GETTING TO THE OTHER SIDE OF VICTORY

———◄•••►———

DONNA HOPKINS

First Printing, 2018.

ISBN: 978-0-9989702-0-2

13th & Joan
500 N. Michigan Avenue, Suite #600
Chicago, IL 606116
Printed in the United States of America.

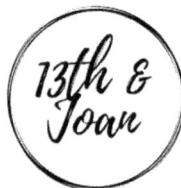

WWW.13THANDJOAN.COM

TESTIMONIES

———◄ ♦ ● ♦ ►———

"Donna's motivation and drive to be the best is very impressive, but what is most impressive is how she lives her life. Her amputation has not slowed her down or kept her down like many people who suffer an amputation. She lives life to the fullest. She is strong, determined, elegant and full of life. I have never seen her down or despondent. She has mentored other patients and is a role model for others that have suffered an amputation. Donna continues to move forward with energy and exuberance."

— Mike Corcoran,
Medical Center Orthotics and Prosthetics (MCOP)

"Donna Hopkins and I both arrived in the National Capital Region in 1983, me as a professional football player and Donna in full pursuit of fulfilling her dreams of becoming both a corporate executive and a sports media personality. While many things have changed over the course of thirty plus years, there is only one thing that my friend Donna has never lost, and that is "The Will to Win!

In her book *Getting to the Other Side of Victory* Donna Hopkins does more than tell her extraordinarily story, she somehow allows each one of us to access the same wind thermals that have helped her to soar to great heights in life, despite tremendous adversity. A must read Indeed!"

— Darrell Green,
Associate Athletic Director,
George Mason University,
Pro Football Hall of Fame

"A woman who gives, inspires and thrives. With grace and a smile, she shares her story — never asking for pity or sympathy and always relying on her faith to help her confront what life has dealt her. You will read not only about her incredible medical journey, but also about how her faith journey has gotten her to the other side of victory. She is driven to always do her best. Her words in *Getting to the Other Side of Victory* will inspire and comfort you. You will get to know a truly great woman."

— Dr. Shawna Willey,
Professor of Surgery at Georgetown University Medical
Center, Director of MedStar's Regional
Breast Health Program

ACKNOWLEDGMENTS

—◀ ◆ ● ◆ ▶—

I never thought that I would become an author; it is indeed an art. It is with much gratitude and abundant awe that I would like to thank everyone who helped me write and publish *Getting to the Other Side of Victory.*

To my biggest support team, who kept me sane throughout the process. I am grateful beyond words for my family and cherished friends. You all are the driving force that has helped to propel me to VICTORY in writing this book.

Thanks to the excellent team of individuals of Wunderlich Kaplan Communications — Gwen Wunderlich, Dara Kaplan, Karolin Kreke and Elif Mamak. It was a pleasure to work with all of you. What a powerhouse. You embodied my mission, the desire to do good in the world and make an impact.

Thanks to the fabulous staff at 13thandjoan for all my publishing needs, with special thanks to Ardre Orie. What a fantastic opportunity it was to work with you. You genuinely understand and make it possible for every author to achieve success in meeting their aspirations.

I am very grateful to Gail Robinson, my first editor, for believing in my storytelling. Thanks to your scrutiny, care and positive reactions to the early drafts of my manuscript, which pushed me to dig deeper into myself to pull out even more.

Many thanks to Diane Cheesebrough for agreeing to be that fine-tuning eye that I needed that gave my story more life. Many thanks to Jarrett Bell for your positive, impactful words of encouragement reading over my manuscript.

To my niece Tequika Tate, who inspired me with her gift of writing. Thanks for your reassurance, support, and guidance in cheering me on. Thank you for pushing me each step of the way and for making me believe in myself as a writer. You saw in me what I didn't see in myself.

Special thanks to Bonnie Burke, who invested in me years ago as my mentor, friend and supporter. She coached and pushed me in the written word, and gave me the courage to believe in my writing abilities. Who knew that years later, I would be an author?

Many thanks to Brian Belts, my graphic designer; what a fantastic book cover, which speaks volumes about the book. Much gratitude to my photographers — Jeff Fowler for that great picture for my book cover, and Yvette Gagnon, who I appreciate for all the times you were there when I needed pictures. Thanks to Karen Hopson, my makeup artist; you are the real deal.

Many thanks to my church family at the Temple of Healing Waters for all of your prayers that speak to this book. I especially thank my Pastor, First Lady, and Church Mom, Dr. Chad Carlton & Darice Carlton, Mother Rena Carlton, and my mentor, Leslie Bishop-Joe.

DEDICATION

———◄ ♦ ● ♦ ►———

o my parents, the late Irving and Nazimova Hopkins, what can I say about two incredible individuals — your strength, your fight, your zeal for life, which I strive to embody.

I especially dedicate Chapter 4, "My Last Walk for a Minute," to Nettie, Lillian, Carolyn, Adrianna, Tequika, Tonitta, Alisha, Nettiel, Dru, Marcy, Annie, Cindy, Thomas, Nicole, Dewayne, Roland, Cory, Sommer, and Leslie Bishop-Joe. You saw it all, and I thank you for allowing me to see all that happened through your eyes as I was out of it most of those 2 ½ months.

I would like to thank all the brilliant individuals at Medical Center Orthotics & Prosthetics (MCOP). I would like to especially thank Mike Corcoran, Ian Fothergill, Art Molnar and Roger Hamilton who pushed the envelope and met me at every challenge. You were the vehicle that gave me hope and provided me with everything that I needed not only to walk again, but proceed with my sporting endeavors and other life occurrences.

To ÖSSUR, if losing my leg had to happen, I'm so glad that you continue to be a trailblazer in pushing forward in the advancement of prosthetics. You are the hope for the amputee community in getting us as close as possible to what we were before. You allow for our dreams to continue. You have answered my every request. I love your energy and passion for what you do. Thanks for your willingness to do everything possible to bring life back into an amputee world. I am tremendously grateful for all that you have done for me and continue to do.

CONTENTS

FOREWORD

———◄ ♦ ♦ ♦ ►———

othing in life is guaranteed. You start out in life visualizing and planning what your life will be 5, 10, 20 years down the line. You govern yourself by the age-old saying that if you fail to plan, then you should plan to fail. So, you plan every detail of your life to a tee. What happens when life changes course unexpectedly, and the plan made is thrown off so severely that you aren't sure how or if you will ever recover?

Getting to the Other Side of Victory is a real demonstration of what happens when life goes from bright hopes to a seemingly dim light in a tunnel. It takes courage, tenacity, and a strong will to fight through some of the most hopeless times, but even more, it takes a God-centered belief and relationship to believe beyond what you can see in your current circumstances. It is so easy to believe the unfavorable reports, thoughts, and commentary that people say to us and that we often tell ourselves. Those things like: "You're never going to make it out of this," "There's no way you can beat this," "Who is ever going to want you after this?" The more you hear it, the easier it becomes to believe it.

These are the very times that we learn exactly who we are and what we are made of, as hard as they may be. For each person, the circumstance will be different, and you should never take what someone else is going through lightly. Your challenge may not be the same as your neighbor's, but for them, it is a challenge all the same. No one knows what it is like to walk in your shoes. No one can tell you how you should feel, and absolutely, no one should tell you when you should be over a "thing." Everyone deserves the right to process their pain, hurt, and disappointment in their own time. But the key is not to make a habit of living in a place of despair.

Life is a very delicate dance. You must know when to stop and deal with your pain, and when to get up and fight. You must learn to study your opponent and its tactics while allowing yourself moments to grieve the unexpected devastation that comes along with your challenge. You must talk yourself out of bed while presenting a smile to cover your pain. Every step you take on your path to victory requires you to stay in step with your opponent.

When going to the other side of victory, you should understand that it may not be a pretty fight. More than likely you are going to walk away with cuts, bruises, and sometimes major scars. You may even walk away feeling disjointed, dismembered, and disconnected at times.

Quite often you will feel like absolutely no one understands your pain and feelings of ugliness. Your instincts will tell you to shut down and retreat within yourself. However, do not be fooled by the tricks of your enemy and opponent. Sure there will be times when you must fight some battles alone, but when you are fighting the war of your life, you need to have your army of support around you.

Life offers you no guarantees, except that you will have a day to check in and a day to check out, what happens in between is all up to you. It's easy to lie down and take the knockout call, but to be a champion, a real champion, you must get up and fight. The victory is not in the bragging rights of not ever being knocked down; it is in the number of times that you get knocked down and then get back up.

Victory comes when you're lying there, and the light keeps blinking off and on, each time staying off longer and longer, and you hear that small still voice say, "Get up! Greater is He that is in you, than He that is in the world. Get up! There is still work to do. Get up! You are more than a conqueror. GET UP, and go to the other side of Victory!"

INTRODUCTION

———◄◆◆►———

Scars there are many; I call them my battle weapons of life. I can look down my entire body and see them all. Some are more pronounced than others; each has its own story to tell. The scars are a reminder of what I've come through and survived.

My journey has been one of peaks and valleys, at times with rivers of tears running down my face and carpet-imprinted knees from the pouring out of prayers that echoed my heartbeat to God, the one that was bottling up my every plea for help.

In years, down the road, each plea would be withdrawn at the most crucial time for my survival. In all the tests and distresses that came my way, what was essential was remembering that my assignment from God was not over yet and I had to get up.

What I realized now was the pivotal importance of why being an athlete was so compelling and captivating to me. My interest in sports began when I was a young child; I used to play flag football with my brothers in our back-yard. My dad had nailed a basketball hoop on the shed in our backyard. My brother's friends from the neighborhood would come over to play. I wanted to participate, but they wouldn't let me. So, when the ball bounced next to me, I would take and keep it until they allowed me to play. Over time we played so much that the once-grassy area was beaten down to dirt.

From there, I had the sports itch. I ran Amateur Athletic Union (AAU) track in middle school, during the summers, and continued running when I got to high school. I also played basketball and a little tennis. I went on to earn schol-arships in both basketball and track.

The thrill of competition ignited my most competitive nature, which in turn would play a significant role in the battles, illnesses, and injuries that I would come to face. My competitive nature aided in my endurance, as it would become the medicine I used to heal myself inside and out and helped me in pushing ahead to whatever life threw my way. However, I knew that the primary medicine was a strong foundation from my parents and a relationship with God, which had been built up in me since childhood. These were the real antidotes and tonics that went through my veins to heal the poison of my life's pains and misfortunes.

The unique result of going through something as incon-ceivable as I did was finding out my identity and my makeup. You never know what is in you until faced with a crisis. I found that God had placed within me an inner fight that would propel me to victory in each battle I had to go through.

Eight years later after the amputation of my left leg, I'm finishing this book, because it gives me a chance to share my road to recovery and what it has taken to climb back into the game of life. Looking through the window of what I went through, I realize that I was in a fight for my life mentally, physically, and spiritually on many occasions. Although I didn't wear my pain on my sleeve for the world to see it didn't mean that there weren't lingering effects. As I looked at my adversities in moving forward, I had to come to grips with the fact that in one's lifetime, some alarming things are going to happen, things which one has no control over. Getting through and working through the brokenness is vital in moving forward to survival, recovery, and victory.

When I processed the difficulties on my journey, it left me with different questions that remained unanswered. I asked God these questions: How does one not quit on life when life seems to have quit on them? How do I put a smile on my face when life's misfortunes and trials have me crying and drowning? How do I keep going when life's ugly blows keep hitting me time and time again like knockout punches?

In 2 Corinthians 4:8-9 (Living Bible), it says, "We are hard pressed on every side by trouble, but not crushed and broken. We are perplexed because we don't know why things happen as they do, but we don't give up and quit. We are hunted down, but God never abandons us. We get knocked down, but we get up again and keep going."

The answer that God gave me is if you can go through the process in whatever you will face in life, know that the skies will clear and you will be able to see the brightness of life again. You must find what it is that will get you to the other side of victory! An article I was reading asked what is it that turns the light back on in your life and brings a smile to your face and joy to your heart? Thinking about that statement, I realized that this is the pathway that one should go down that will lead them to victory.

In 1997, 1999, 2009, and 2010, I found myself sinking into the depths of unknown waters. I had breast cancer twice, thyroid disease and the amputation of part of my left leg, each time having to face extreme adversities. Somehow, I found a way to climb back into the lifeboat to make it over to the other side of victory.

As I retrace the steps of my journey, I'm hoping that those reading this book may gain insight, hope, and encouragement on how they too can be not just a warrior, but an overcomer in moving forward through whatever they face. Know that the unthinkable life storms and tragedies one faces do not have to destroy your tomorrow. There is a remedy to whatever the situation may be. Life does not have to be lived forever in pain. Don't spend a lifetime counting and watching the storms in your life—learn to enjoy the sun when it does come out and shine!

1
BATTLE SCARS

———◄♦●♦►———

It is during our darkest moments that we must focus to see the light.
— Aristotle

G lancing back at my childhood, I had a very adventurous spirit. I recall these words from my parents time and time again: "I told you not to do that, and you did it anyway." There was always a price to pay, whether at the hands of my parents or at the hands of life itself. Either way, it was a lesson in life that would no doubt further build toward my life's comebacks.

To understand my later sufferings, I search my childhood memories. I remember receiving the first scar at the hands of an old washing machine. I hadn't started school yet, and I remember being out on the back porch of our home in Winona, West Virginia. My mom was washing clothes in her early model wringer washing machine. It had a huge round base with wooden rollers that sat on top to wring the water out of the clothes as you removed them from the machine. A tin tub on a wooden bench behind the base of the machine was there to catch the clothing from my mom's hands. As I watched with intrigued eyes, my small hands wanted to put clothes on the two wooden rollers to assist my mom or to appease my curiosity. She had repeatedly told me not to mess with the washing machine, but I was just waiting for the right opportunity.

As my mom gathered the clothing to hang on a line, I decided this was my opportunity to help her. As soon as she went out into the yard and down the hillside, I tried to put a sock through the wringer, and it got tangled around the rollers. As I tried to retrieve and pinch at a portion of the sock, my hand got pulled through the rollers. I screamed out for dear life.

My mom dropped the basket of clothing and ran back up the hillside toward me. By the time she reached me, my right arm had gone through the rollers to my elbow. My mom jerked the machine's power cord out of the socket and started beating the handle of the top portion of the rollers like a mad woman. It was an intense fight between her and the washing machine because they both wanted my arm.

Fortunately for me, she eventually won that battle over my arm but lost the war as she ended up breaking the machine to free my arm. I stood there in tears, with my arm battered and bruised from the war that was just caused by my own doing. The only thing that saved me from getting my behind beaten was my injured arm and my beseeching quest for affection from my mom. Even today, when I look at my arm, I can see the almost-faded imprint of the battle that took place on my right arm many years ago.

As I got a little older, the washing machine incident proved to be a lesson that I didn't learn well. My sense of discovery almost made me come face-to-face with death.

My dad and mom had gone to the store, and they left my two younger sisters and me under the watchful care of our older brothers and sisters. They were supposed to make sure we didn't get into any trouble; I must say they didn't do the best job. A jolt of electricity almost collided with me, and the result would not have been in my favor. Death almost called my name.

I was around ten, and we were still living in Winona. I was out on our front porch. I had picked up an old baton and was just messing around. My oldest sister Lillian, who was in high school at the time, was a majorette in the band. I was always twirling her baton with the vision of myself one day stepping high in that majorette uniform.

The light fixture on the porch was missing the light bulb, and I kept looking up at it. My curiosity made me want to stick one end of the baton in the socket. It was like lightning hit when I jabbed it up in the socket, and it blew the baton right out of my hands. It also knocked out the power through the entire house.

My brothers and sisters came running to see what happened. I stood there mystified, too young and dumb to realize that I had just escaped death. I was lucky to be alive, and I welcomed the scolding that was coming my way from all parties. The end of the baton was burnt and black from the tip all the way down to the base of the metal. The only thing that saved me from seeing the pearly gates that evening was the rubber tip that was in my hand on the other end of the baton. Fortunately for us, we got the power back on before my parents arrived back home.

However, no one had to say anything because the burnt edges of the light fixture revealed what had happened. The only thing that kept me from having a sore behind again was my near-death experience, but it didn't save me from the tongue-lashing my Dad gave me, which was far worse than a whipping.

Later, we moved from Winona to a neighborhood in Oak Hill, West Virginia, known as Harlem Heights. I was now in the fifth grade. Again, my parents, with these catchy phrases, used to tell us "a hard head makes a soft behind." For me, this time might have been a good time to have a hard head. Without even being aware, I was headed down the road to becoming an athlete. My sense of competitiveness kicked into gear and led me to my next injury.

I thought that I would try my hand at broad jumping from a tree limb. There was an enormous tree between our house and Annie's, my first friend in our new neighborhood. She, along with my brother Tony and my younger sister Nettie, used to climb up this tall, broad, full tree. It had some of the best limbs for climbing and hanging upside down. We used to go to the top as far as we could climb and just sit and talk, looking down at everything that surrounded us below and outward. It was also an excellent place to hide from my parents.

Getting up the tree was somewhat of a challenge for our small frames, however.

Although I had long legs to help me, I still had to swing myself up from the long bottom trunk. I had done this many times, propelling myself up like a gymnast, and then hanging upside down like I was on the uneven parallel bars. I was fortunate that day that my dad had just laid dirt down under this tree; otherwise, I probably would have broken my neck. Annie, Nettie, and I were trying to see who could broad jump the farthest by swinging from the branch of the tree limb outward to the ground. My competitive nature wasn't about to let me lose this challenge.

It had rained earlier that day, and the branches were wet. When I got up to swing, my hands slipped from the branch and the next thing I remember, I was telling my brother Larry to put me down. I had been knocked out by the fall, but only for a few seconds, so I was told. My mom made me go in and lie down on her bed, but my headache just got worse. My dad arrived home from work, and I was grateful that his concern for me was far more significant than him giving me the Irving "you in-trouble-look" or his severe vocal blasting, which I probably deserved, especially since he had warned us so often to stay out of that tree.

I had a concussion and ended up in the hospital for a few days. It was my first hospital stay, and I hoped my last. The funny thing is, I thought I had escaped discipline for my actions but they came back to haunt me once I was out of the hospital. I don't know if getting my buns sizzled would have been better because I got my dad's vocal thrashing after my brain and thoughts had mended themselves back together.

Growing up, I never saw my frequent injuries as being dominant or something that I couldn't survive, probably because I was too young or clueless to really understand their magnitude. I just kept getting up from them. Those childhood injuries toughened me up and allowed me to develop an inner strength. In many ways, those injuries told me a lot about myself: I don't like to lose.

I also understood my adventurous spirit and competitive nature, because, when it came to sports, sports matched up with my temperament. Every injury suffered as a child build resilience, which was the driving force that pushed me to become the best athlete that I would become later in life.

The most devastating and shattering wound of my childhood, for my family and me, came when I was fifteen. My parents, most of my siblings, and I had gone to a Bible study at our old church in Winona that day. When we returned, my dad was wondering why my brother Tony was not back home yet. He worked cutting people's lawns in various nearby communities and had gone out in our dad's red pickup truck before we left. My dad went out looking for him but was unable to locate him.

Sad to say, we later found out what had happened to Tony while watching the local nightly news. There Tony's body was, lying stretched out on the roadside, uncovered and exposed like he was rubbish; his body showing signs of the trauma he had experienced. What a piercing sight to see on the news and to learn of his death that way. How callous.

You can imagine the jolt and hurt we all felt at that moment. In a state of shock and disbelief, the life was sucked out of all of us.

Tony, a year older than me, had been killed in a truck accident at the age of 16. He was on the highway about 10 minutes from home and had hit a wall coming onto the ramp heading home, we were told. The accident report said that Tony had hit his head on the front windshield and was thrown from the truck. He died instantly. Another person who was in the truck with him had lived.

I didn't know how to handle his death, so I was mad at him for dying. I blamed him because I didn't understand and had no one else to blame. It was like I thought that Tony could do something about it, so I said, "That is what he gets," as if he did something to deserve death. It was crazy.

I still hurt today, because I told God he took Tony's life too early and it wasn't fair. Tony didn't even get a chance to live.

During his wake, I remember my dad taking my sister Nettie and me to see his body. We both were putting on brakes, resisting as he pushed us forward to look at Tony's body. His dark fingernails drew my eyes to them. I don't even know if I looked up at his face after seeing the coldness and emptiness of his nails. From that moment, I told myself I would never view another person's body again after that experience. Their lifeless and unmoving body was not the last thing I wanted to remember about anybody.

This experience made me ponder life after death, and how others will remember us. At Tony's funeral, I listened as people talked about his nature, his kind-heartedness and other compelling things about his character and the kind of person he was. I thought to myself; I hope they said this to his face while he was living. We all tend to make these comments after someone is gone.

Moving forward was painful. Memories can be a good and bad reminder. Silently I had to come to grips with how to handle Tony's death. I was feeling everyone else's pain while trying to escape my own. No one was saying anything.

As a family, we never talked about Tony's death openly. I don't know if anyone knew what to say; I didn't. I believe that all of us were hiding away in our silent pain and disbelief, each trying to handle it in our own way. Talking about it only stirred up the anxiety; asking questions would yield no answers to the why.

As for my parents and my siblings, this was all new to us, and no one knew how to or could take the lead in coping with Tony's death. It was hard for everyone. For my dad and mom, you could see the distress, hurt and emptiness on their face, even though they try to hide it from us. You could sense it by the quietness of the house. I never saw them cry, but I'm sure they did when they could escape and let out what they were honestly feeling.

We each had to become our own grief counselor, pulling on God and his word for whatever we needed. All of us knew enough about God and now was the time to trust God as a family, and individually. To trust God in the light when all is well is nothing, but this was the time when we had to trust God in the darkness.

From this tragedy and anguish, I was getting a lesson of strength, stamina, and courage by watching my parents and how they went through and survived Tony's death. The strength that I saw in both parents after losing a child was remarkable, but pushing through it for their other children was a testimony of fortitude. I believe that if they had to pick a scripture from the Bible, one would be from Isaiah 41:10: "Do not fear, for I am with you; do not be dismayed, for I am your God. I will strengthen you and help you; I will uphold you with my righteous right hand."

They say we can look back at our childhood and see how it has shaped our lives. I believe my first scars, battle wounds, and losses later helped me handle the things that were yet to come.

2

MY DNA

————◄◆◆►————

As we rise to meet the challenges that are a natural part of living, we awaken to our many undiscovered gifts, to our inner power and our purpose.
— Susan L. Taylor

headed to West Virginia over Mother's Day weekend in 2013. This trip was necessary for so many reasons. It was the first time back home since my mom passed away in 2011, following my dad's death in 2009. My brothers and sisters who had left West Virginia dreaded going home, more now since both parents were deceased. Although two of my sisters still lived there, going back for me felt like finding one's bearing and a connection in a strange land. It was the perfect time to revisit the first place I called home, to reconnect and find healing and purpose since I had been through so much.

I made the five-hour trip alone, which was therapeutic for me. It gave me and my thoughts the needed time to be free from the rat race of processing too much data in a busy work week, among all the other things pulling at me and my time. However, I still didn't like making that drive home on WV I-64, not with the long stretch of highway, and steep mountains with winding roads that made it feel like you were on the world's most dangerous roller coaster ride.

I arrived home to the surprise of two of my sisters, Carolyn and Adrianna. Although they were happy to see me, they seemed baffled as to why I was there.

As I walked through the house, it gave me an empty feeling. My childhood house that once was filled with all kinds of traffic was now a quiet vessel for former travelers passing through from time to time.

As I stood in the living room, my eyes gravitated over to the couch. It made me think about my mom; I could see her there in her last year alive. The living room had become her living quarters, although her bedroom was just a few steps away. She felt more content on the couch, not wanting to be closed off in her room. Her health had deteriorated to where she was no longer able to walk or care for herself, and you could see the pain in her eyes, not wanting to be a burden to anyone. It was hard for me to see her that way, knowing the rock she had been to all of us for so many years. In her last year alive, we became the pillar of strength for her.

My eyes then were drawn to the area of my dad's big, comfortable, oversized blue reclining chair that most of us ran to when we came home. It was his favorite chair after he had a stroke in 2008. When I came back for visits, that is where I would find him sitting for extended hours during the day.

As I took it all in, my thoughts and heart were at a loss to recover the one-time joy of home. I fought back the tears, trying not to let my two sisters see my emotions.

The next morning, I got started early. I only had a short window and much to do and see in the brief period before leaving on Sunday morning. I was off to unite the past and the present.

I gathered the directions from one of my sisters because the way to get to our first home in Winona had changed so much over the years with all the new highways, bridges and shortcuts. I was trying to envision how to get there in my head, but I was still confused. Adrianna saw the puzzled look on my face and decided to just go with me.

Winona, West Virginia is a small town in the Appalachian Mountains, with beautiful rolling foothills and breathtaking views, which none of us paid much attention when growing up there.

As we got closer to the town, some of the sites and places started to come back to my memory, and I could see us as children moving about. The look of the area was different; it was like the town I knew had vanished. I had not been back to this area for at least 30 years since we moved when I was very young. The only thing that was still visible was a small pathway leading up the hill to where our house once stood.

Much of what I recalled was gone; the church I once attended with my siblings had been torn down and replaced by a large trailer court. The only store and post office in the community was now a burned frame. The elementary school I attended in my first few years was still standing, but it was now an old building not even resembling a school. The wooden bridge that we crossed over to get to the school was still there but was now a decaying structure. My sister pointed out how the dirt road that once led up to my aunt's house and other homes — once surrounded by trees that hid their homes — was now a clear-cut view, exposing everything. It was like that area, and the town had been undressed and bared.

As we continued to drive through the area, I recalled what it once looked like and the sounds of life and living that once echoed throughout this small region.

I could see our house that stood at the top of two hills, overlooking houses down below. It was a mature white farmhouse, two stories with great character. The countryside and the panoramic view of homes running alongside the hills rendered an incredible backdrop of breathtaking views of a small town that once was full of life. I searched my thoughts as my eyes took in the emptiness of what was no longer there. However, growing up there, it speaks to my foundation, which was built on the simple things in life and cultivated on developing my uniqueness. Seeing the area allows me to identify and unveil my strength through my early experiences. It also gave me a greater appreciation in understanding the beauty of the simplicity of family and how important family became down through the years for me.

Before we made our way out of the town, we stopped by the area where the church once stood. Growing up, my parents instilled strong Christian values into all our lives. Going to church as a child wasn't a choice you made on your own, not in our house. As a young child, each Sunday morning we would all get up and, most times, walked to church, although my dad drove. We enjoyed walking as we engaged in our surroundings and entertained ourselves before getting to church. We knew that once we entered the church doors, there was no more playing around, not if you wanted peace later. There were many reasons why we loved walking to church; it had more to do with our journey back home afterward. We would stop by the little town store and get candy with some of the money we were supposed to put in the church offering. We made sure to dispose of all the evidence of our tasty delights before we reached home.

The church consisted of a few people from the neighborhood, but mainly my relatives on my dad's side and a few on my mom's. My mom attended a church in a nearby town called Ansted where she grew up. I remember her being involved in many church affairs and doing special events where we would join her. Most of my siblings and I attended my dad's church, where he was a deacon and the treasurer.

I was baptized as a young child in the church pool that was stationed outside in front of the church. I had accepted Jesus Christ into my life as my Lord and savior. Over the years, it wasn't just about going to church for me, but rather about developing a personal relationship with God. I desired to have the heart of God.

The heart speaks to who you are; it embodies the womb of your character. I started to understand what that meant for my life. I thought about how important church was to my family as I grew up in our household and how that foundation would be essential to me as I faced so much in my early years and moving forward. It is those morals and values that were instilled in me by both parents and the personal attributes that guide me and make me who I am.

As I look back and remember my mom, there are so many things I can pull from. But what resonates in my mind are those earlier years as a child that touch me most profoundly.

One experience was when I was young, and my mom was washing my sisters' and my hair. She had her hands full when it came to washing our hair — four girls, one after the other, with long natural hair, and she didn't even have a sink. She washed our hair in a tin basin out on our back porch during the summer. By the time she finished washing my hair, it was like I had been in a tug of war, me crying because soap got into my eyes, and her giving me whiplash combing my hair out. There was one style after you got your hair washed, five plaits, one on the top, two on the side, and two in the back. There was nothing stylish or attractive about that hairdo. You loathed getting your hair washed during that time, but laugh about it all now. Part of me yearns to have those special moments back.

My mom had this incredible strength. You could see it through all that she had endured. She had a supernatural force that I'm sure she didn't even realize was powerful to all who were onlookers. Over the years, I watched as she overcame various illnesses time and time again. I drew on that, and I'm stronger, tougher, and more resilient because of her. Most of all, I found the strength to withstand countless challenges on my own. Her DNA spilled into my bloodstream with an overcoming spirit that made me solid.

I believe that I became a better person from my dad's strict rules and discipline. He grounded, molded and shaped me into the person I am today. I think that I'm a better person because of him. When my dad was calling on me and my sister Nettie to help him with what I considered work, I later realized that it was him getting to know us and our individuality.

When I was around 10, there was no such thing as being afraid or escaping the disgusting acts of cruelty that would later become our dinner.

My dad had gone hunting and brought back some rabbits and squirrels he had killed. Nettie and I were called to help him take off the skin. As I stood there gazing at my dad, I wanted to be anywhere but there. I had one end of the animal while my dad had the other end. I held on while he cut around the middle part of the body, which helped us get a grip on the animal's skin.

I was a skinny child, and while my dad pulled on one end, I was clasping my end, trying to keep a foothold to support my position. I didn't want to end up on the ground with my face punching into the rabbit or squirrel. The reward for us at the end was the lucky rabbit's foot or the squirrel tail that we attached to the ends of our bike handlebars.

Despite the farm animals, rabbits, squirrels, chicken and other things that my dad would engage me in, there were moments of enjoyment when it came to working beside him. Nettie, Adrianna and I used to ride in the back of my dad's red pickup truck around the mountains, although we never thought about how dangerous it was at the time. With our mouths open, we let the wind from the speed of the truck echo sounds out. We would let the wind hit our faces to take in the fresh mountain air and feel the power of the air gliding across our faces. It was like we were on a thrill ride, waiting to throw our hands up to enjoy the full effects of the ride.

Sometimes when it was cold, we would get close to the bed of the truck so that we could shield ourselves from the wind and other elements. On most of these trips we were going to our grandmother's house, my dad's mom. Before we arrived at her house, my dad would stop to allow us to get a taste of water running down off the rocks of the mountainside. We would scoop it up in our hands as our mouths took in the refreshing coldness of the water. Once we finished getting water, we jumped back into the truck and proceeded to cross a two-car bridge. I hated crossing that bridge because it was such a tight squeeze for two cars.

You could almost reach out and give high fives to people in other vehicles coming across.

Driving around the mountains with those curvy roads was no treat for me, by the time we reached our destination, my head was reeling and what was inside my stomach wanted to be released.

My grandmother welcomed seeing us. We would visit her quite often because we worked alongside my dad in the garden he had planted for her. He seemed to believe it was a daughter-and-father bonding time working with him in the garden. He saw this as spending time with us; we saw it as being dinner for mosquitoes. Sometimes Nettie and I would sneak away to indulge in some other activity.

During those visits, we would quickly take off our shoes and gingerly walk barefoot on the gravel down to the one-room Post Office. We stayed off the pavement because the surface was too hot. On our way back, we would stop along the roadside to pick and eat raspberries and strawberries until our bellies were satisfied. Before we headed back to our grandmother's house, we would cross over to my uncle's house to climb and eat off his cherry tree. By the time we ran back to my grandmother's house; it was time for us to jump back into the truck to head home.

Although I had ten siblings, I thought about Nettie's and my relationship over time. She and I had an unspeakable rapport. Everyone always thought that we were twins and my mom made it believable by dressing us alike all the time.

Nettie and I have always experienced life's wonders together. She and I are a strong rope for each other to pull on. It is a unique bond that started as children and has deepened. As kids, we did everything together. Although I had other siblings, it was like Nettie and I just connected, our spirits spoke the same language at a young age. I remember as small children having to share a twin bed with her. At times we would fight because we felt like one of us was taking too much of the bed. Later, when we moved to Harlem Heights, we shared a room. I was in the top twin bunk bed, while she had the lower one. Sometimes after watching the scary vampire show "Dark Shadows," when Nettie went to sleep I would check her neck to make sure she hadn't gotten bitten. We played in the band together, had some of the same friends, had our first job together, went to the same college, ran track in both high school and college and ended up moving to the same area as adults.

It wasn't until high school that we become more than just sisters. We became each other's cheerleader, fighter, supporter, best friend, as a more significant appreciation developed. Although we are unique individuals, it's as though our souls are one. The broad admiration for each other and the bond over time has never died.

For my other siblings, each of us had our particular kind of relationship because of the age difference growing up. There are about five of us close in age; we were more connected because we just did more things together. However, my 2010 amputation created a closer-knit connection with

Carolyn, one of my sisters who is a few years older, as she spent countless hours with me at the hospital. Something happened; I believe that we both came to understand each other's nature even more.

During my time at home, I thought about friendships and how my closest friendships today formed when I moved into our new neighborhood in Harlem Heights. We were all pretty much around the same age, and it was through our first job at a church center that our friendships started, grew and became enriched when we all ended up at the same college.

The Hilltop Baptist Center was where we all had our first job; Marcy, Annie, my sister Nettie and me. Although we didn't get paid much and worked long hours for about three summers together, it was those summers that bonded us all for life. A few highlights of those summer work days at the Baptist building were the snack bar. It was a place that ended our work day by being treated to the item of our choice; which, most times, was a homemade milkshake that we all delighted in after everyone else was gone.

Then it was the canoes for the camp sessions. One day Annie and I decided that we would take one out, two non-swimmers without permission and no one there to help if we turned over.

We dragged a canoe to the edge of the pond, turned it over in the water and proceeded to climb in. However, before we could get our bodies in the canoe, it turned over with us halfway in it. We both were petrified, struggling and kicking to get our balance and stand up. Once we could, we hurried out of the water.

We pulled the canoe out of the water and placed it halfway back in the area we had found it. Wet and still looking startled, we ran to the main building so that we could dry off before the Pastor returned. Good thing we were only in knee-deep water; otherwise it wasn't going to be a good outcome for us.

There was also the tarry in the night when we were scared out of our wits. We were all in the basement in our room, clowning around and telling scary stories while service was finishing up, but before we had to head to the snack bar for our final work duty.

Someone knocked on the door. Annie shouted out. "Who's there?" But no one answered. They knocked again. Annie said, "I'm going to put my fist through the door." We opened the door to look out, but no one was there, so we went down the hallway, one by one. Suddenly someone jumped out of an opening. We all took off running in a panic. Someone had bumped into me and almost knocked me down, but I kept moving. I was on my hands-and-knees bent over running and ran right over Nettie until I could get up straight fully.

We all ran to the kitchen on the second floor and went out on the platform still shaking, with a terrified look on our faces. We started shouting at each other about what had happened. One person stayed behind and hidden and said it was the administrator, but we didn't believe her.

We jumped down from the platform and headed toward the front of the building. When we got to the front of the building the administrator came out and was laughing. We didn't see the humor.

One summer, a male missionary had come to the center for part of their mission. We had gotten to know him over the summer. One day, since we didn't have anything going on at the center, we talked him into letting us drive his car on the property. With the administrator gone, it was perfect. None of us had drivers' licenses yet, but we figured no harm since we weren't going out on the highway.

Nettie just watched from the side (she decided not to engage in this venture), but for the others, it was too tempting for us to pass up. We were on a dirt road that went around part of the property next to the pond area. One person got behind the wheel, while the other two jumped in the back seat, with the missionary on the passenger's side telling us what to do before we started up the car. Annie and I took it easy, putting a little gas on the pedal when we got up to drive, but the last person thought that she was the only car out on an open roadway. She took off, and all you could see was a cloud of dust behind us. The dirt road was bumpy and uneven with dips, and because she was going too fast, we were bouncing around from side to side in the back seat. We were laughing and enjoying every moment of the ride. The missionary told her to slow down and decided that our driving classes were over. We all headed back to the main building, sworn to secrecy.

From the Baptist Center in our earlier days, we each one by one ended up at the same college, first Marcy, then Annie, me and lastly Nettie. We all were roommates for a few years living in Moran Hall; Nettie and Marcy were roommates, as were Annie and me. It was our road trips back to Fairmont State College that were interesting. One time we got stopped by the police for speeding. The officer asked Marcy, the driver, to roll down the window; she only cracked it a little enough to give him her license. He kept asking her to turn it down more, again she only rolled it down about an inch or so. Once we could leave, we all were laughing so hard.

Throughout our childhood, college days and long after them all, we are not only friends but family.

When I look at my friendships, they are one of life's greatest treasures; there is something about how people touch your heart, your soul, and they are forever a part of you. My long-lasting friendships with Marcy, Annie, Cindy, and Nettie is a sisterhood that has been cultivated over the years by our willingness, dedication, and support of each other; whether slightly miles or cities apart we are forever connected and linked.

After college, we all ended up in the Washington, D.C. metropolitan area. When one of us moved to the area and needed a place to stay, we were there for each other with open doors. I remember a time when I needed to move from a house I was renting, and Marcy was leaving the area, she offered her condo to me for months, free. There was one time that I injured my knee playing basketball, and by the time I reached the hospital, Nettie, Cindy, and Annie were there. One year, hearing that one of Marcy's children was sick, it was nothing for me to get on a plane and head there for support.

We have become Aunties to each other's children and were there for graduations, school activities, injuries, and illnesses. We all traveled to California twice for two of Marcy's children's high school graduations; while we were celebrating their accomplishments, it was more of a reunion for us. We have laughed at situations no matter how tragic, frustrating or confusing; cried together from broken relationships; and celebrated each other's successes. I have been truly blessed to have wonderful and amazing friends. My aces have had a profound impact on my life. Our lives have taken many turns, but here we are still with emotional support for each other, being each other's biggest cheerleaders, and being that person who, when we need our handheld most, would come to the rescue.

As I returned to revisit the first place I called home, I allowed my mind to take me back to recall my childhood step by step. What I gathered from each undertaking was a building block and the components that I now realize prepared me and gave me strength and the potency to take on life's suffering, pains, and misfortunes, in not giving up.

3
BETRAYED FROM WITHIN

———◄◆◆►———

Faith is taking the first step even when you don't see the whole staircase.
— Martin Luther King, Jr.

t's January 1997: I'm attending a revival at my church in Maryland. Each year we had spiritual renewal services, a chance to start fresh from whatever you wanted to purge from your life. Little did I know just how important this one would be for me. One night at the revival, I had gotten into a prayer line along with many others.

The person leading the revival was considered a prophet, a person who speaks by divine inspiration, a messenger from God. When he began to pray for me, he said, "Think not that it is strange what you are going to go through." He went on to say, "You are going to be on a platform and able to reach people that I won't be able to." At that point, I stood there trying to process what he was saying and what it meant. My mind wandered to me being in sports broadcasting, and I thought maybe that was it. Then he went on to say that I would need to be like a tree planted by the water. Now I was perplexed.

That night when I got home, I picked up my Bible, as I recalled a passage in the Bible talking about trails and a tree planted by the water. In 1 Peter 4:12 it states, "Beloved, think it not strange concerning the fiery trial, which is to try you, as though some strange thing happened unto you." Then I looked at Jeremiah 17:8, where it states, "He is like a tree planted by water, that sends out its roots by the stream, and does not fear when heat comes, for its leaves remain green, and is not anxious in the year of drought, for it does not cease to bear fruit." Even reading these passages, I still had no idea what it meant to me. I put it in the back of my mind and didn't wrestle with it anymore.

In March of that year, I was sitting at work during the early part of the day. I had touched the top area of my chest, and to my surprise, I felt a raised area on my right breast. Alarmed, I immediately thought to myself; please don't let it be the big C (cancer). I sat there quietly, my mind racing. I was scared, to the point that I didn't want to touch the area again to confirm what I felt.

When you think about cancer, nothing good comes to mind. Most associate it with a death sentence; I did not allow my mind to take me there. As I left work, I said nothing to anyone. I went to the gym for my regular workout; I was trying to keep my mind busy and from the thought of cancer. When I got home later that day, like most, fear arose. Not wanting to alarm my family or close friends, I called no one that evening.

At the time, I was only 36, a fit, healthy person; I wasn't even thinking about mammograms or anything else associated with cancer. When I got up the following morning, I called my primary doctor and informed her about the lump. I'm so glad that breast cancer was being talked about a lot then because I was well informed about the disease, which made me act immediately. Who knows how long the lump had been there; it was just now manifesting itself. Until I could get in to see my primary doctor, it was about staying positive and not allowing my mind to take me to an unwanted diagnosis of my making. Eventually, when I did see my doctor, she had me wait about a month to see if it was associated with my monthly blues or my "unwanted party," as two of my younger nieces described it. In the waiting stage, to keep my mine tranquil and out of distress mode, I tried to go about my business as usual, like nothing was going on.

My follow-up appointment with my doctor revealed that the lump was still there. The thought of cancer now weighed heavily on my mind. She informed me that she was sending me to see a breast surgeon who could better evaluate the lump. Now it was time to tell someone, but not my mom. She was too sick herself and going through her war of getting better in so many ways.

I decided not to tell most of my siblings. I knew they would spill the beans to her because some of them can't hold water. The selective few were ones that I knew could get a prayer through. They also had to be on the same page as I, knowing that I was going to beat cancer if that is what it turned out to be. When you are in a fight for your life, you must have the right people in your corner. The last thing that I needed was people crying more than me. So, I only told my close friends, Annie, Marcy, Cindy, and Nettie, as well as some people from my church and those I needed to inform at my job.

As I walked into the breast care center for my initial consultation with the surgeon, I put on a good face. He had a gentle persona and what settled my mind somewhat was his 30-plus years of experience. Although I did not know at this point if it was cancer, I was looking for answers from him about a dreaded disease that had likely inserted itself into my body. His face was as reassuring as it could be, although he didn't know much yet without doing more tests. As I gathered my speeding thoughts, he performed an ultrasound, which revealed the size of the lump. Still not clear what it was yet, my next appointment would be with radiology to get the clamp-down mammogram that, up until this point, I had only heard people talk about, and their experiences never left me with a good feeling. I wasn't ready for it and even less ready for what it might reveal.

Upon my first mammogram visit, my eyes searched the other women's faces. They either were waiting to go in, as

I was, or for the results of their mammogram tests. Either way, they had a look of disquiet on their face. As they called my name, I entered the room.

My eyes were immediately drawn to the mammogram machine. The unit was huge. I studied it inch-by-inch, focused on the middle frame where it had two transparent plastic plates connected, but separated in the middle. Asking questions, I found out that they were designed to hold and compress the breast in position to see the images at different angles.

As they got started, a cover was placed on the lower half of my body to protect it from the radiation. The technician stood me in front of the x-ray machine, putting my right breast on the platform that held the x-ray film. She then adjusted the position of the platform to match my height, along with positioning my head, arms, and torso so that there was an unobstructed view of my right breast. Once I was in position, she activated the x-ray machine.

Suddenly, the machine imprisoned my right breast and it was trapped between the two clear plastic paddles. The compression was firm. I felt like my entire body went into distress, as I tried to soak up the pain. The technician kept gradually compressing my breast, asking me to hold very still and not to breathe for a few seconds while they took the x-ray, to reduce the possibility of a blurred image. I wanted to yank my breast out of that machine. Who in their right mind thought that they should be putting your breast through that kind of agony? There had to be a better system. Breasts were never supposed to be flat; there is a reason God made them round.

When the examination was complete, the technician asked me to go back to the waiting room until the radiologist could determine if more images were necessary. I was admittedly hoping that wasn't the case.

After a while, the radiologist came back in the room to talk to me. The radiologist stated that the doctor reviewing my film determined that more tests were needed. If you could visualize my face, the worry was written all over it. I tried to read their faces and gather the tone in their voices.

They told me that they saw some calcification deposits — calcium deposits within breast tissue — which was suspicious and they felt that more testing was necessary. A third mammogram was needed, which would show magnification views or a breast biopsy.

Now came all the questions.

They asked me if I had a family history of breast cancer, and at the time the only person I knew of who had a history of breast cancer was one aunt on my mom's side. There were many other health issues on both my dad's and mom's sides, but cancer was not one of them, to the best of my knowledge. Regarding the risk factors for breast cancer, I knew that I ate right and wasn't overweight by any means because of my workout regimen. In fact, I prided myself on taking care of my body. I had done my part, I told myself.

In April, everything became clear; I discovered what the prophecy meant. The prophet had said at the revival, "Think not that it is strange what you are going to go through, but you must be like a tree planted by the water," so I went back to the Bible verses in Peter and Jeremiah again. 1 Peter 4:12 says: "Beloved, think it not strange concerning the fiery trial, which is to try you, as though some strange thing happened unto you." And Jeremiah 17:8: "He is like a tree planted by water, that sends out its roots by the stream, and does not fear when heat comes, for its leaves remain green, and is not anxious in the year of drought, for it does not cease to bear fruit." It simply meant that my roots — my faith — had to go deep down in trusting God.

To further understand those Bible verses, I thought about plants and their root systems. To understand the root system, I did some research; it noted that the root system is a below-ground structure that serves primarily to anchor the plant in the soil and take up water and minerals. The growth and branches of a plant will only be healthy if the roots are strong and profound, the same as a tree. I thought about a palm tree, which can grow in the most desert-like conditions. In times of drought everything around it will dry up and die, but the palm tree will continue to grow in freshness.

As I studied this further, I learned the reason why a palm tree can withstand a storm or a drought is that its long roots go deep down into the ground and reach the water beneath. Along with the depth of a tree root, the roots also spread out wide; most can occupy an area four to seven times the diameter of the crown of the tree.

A tree is only as strong as its roots, so in the illustration of God, who is the soil of our life, He produces the rich minerals and the vitamins that we need to build strong roots, which is our soul, mind, will, and emotions.

The real test of our temperament, spirit, and outlook is our ability to remain standing in the storm, even as we look at the devastation from the storm. What did this mean for me? It meant that I had to let my faith go deep down in God and His word. I had to do what I had been living after all these years, trusting God.

At this moment, I was trying not to focus on the disease that was threatening to rip away my peace and wipe out my joy. What I had to concentrate on in my despair was that, even during this hostile storm in my life, my faith had to stretch deep down in God where I could remain strong, immovable and grounded. Job 14:7 states, "For there is hope for a tree if it is cut down, that it will sprout again, and that its shoots will not cease."

So, in God's promise and my trust in Him, like the tree planted by the water, no matter what the circumstances surrounding me; if it were cancer, I would be renewed and continue to grow and flourish and produce good fruits. No matter what the condition or under the direst of circumstances, I would withstand the hit.

As a believer, I find it funny that we are always telling others that God is a Healer, a Provider, and a Way Maker. But do we believe what we say to others when we find ourselves faced with a situation or in a storm? Sometimes, I think that God wants to see if we believe what we so often preach to others. In looking at what I was facing, I told individuals that God allowed the lump to come up; otherwise, not being at the age to get mammograms, cancer could have grown and probably spread. I realized that the lump coming up saved my life. I also recognized in the midst of this unwanted storm that God was yet in control of what was happening in my life, and therefore it gave me hope.

On June 10, 1997, I had a needle/wire localization biopsy, which would allow my surgeon to evaluate the lump that was visible on my mammogram. The wire localization, which is also known as needle localization, is done by the surgeons to map the route to the mass for the surgical biopsy. To locate the abnormality, they use a mammography technique. The radiologist uses a small needle with a guided wire that they positioned within the breast mass. Once the wire was in place, a mammogram would be performed to verify the position of the wire.

Leading up to the needle localization, I had worked myself up a little because all I could envision was them putting a needle through my skin with the thread at the end. That took me back to my days of sewing, and all I could see was the needle on the sewing machine going through the fabric. As I waited to go into the procedure room, I still was thinking about that needle going through my skin and me being a piece of fabric.

The first thing I noticed when entering the room was the machine with the needle. I checked it out and wondered how the tech was going to get my breast into that machine. I had waited for what seemed like hours, uneasy about the procedure. Finally, the radiologist came in and explained the process before getting started. The first part of the procedure, they would do at the ambulatory building. The tech positioned my body into the machine like they did when I got the mammogram. My face was sideways up against a clear plastic glass, and my right arm placed on the part of the machine. My breast was placed in an area of the machine to insert the needle. The stick from the needle was more like a pinch. Following the wire localization, the tech escorted me to the hospital for surgery.

In June, as I waited for the results, I had plans to run in the Race for the Cure for breast cancer over the weekend, a 5K I had run for 15 years with my sister, Nettie. My doctor was going to have the results early in the next week.

As we stood at the starting line of the race with thousands of people, this time it had a different feel. I looked around, taking it all in as I hid behind my sunglasses; trying to fight back the tears and attempting not to let my emotions overtake me. I wouldn't even talk much to Nettie because the floodgates would have opened and not stopped.

Standing there, I knew that I was running for myself this time. As the gun sounded, I took off. Throughout the race, as Nettie and I had done in previous years, we would look over at each other and ask, "Are you all right?" We were making sure that we helped each other get to the finish line, but that year I told her I was pushing ahead. That June in 1997, I ran and had the best time that I ever had running in the race. In some way, I had set the tone for the march ahead of me, to the process of winning the battle against cancer — if it turned out to be cancer — but in my heart, I already knew that it was.

That Monday, after the race, as I prepared to get my results, one of my best friends, Annie, decided to go with me to my appointment. She probably knew, like me, that the results were not going to be in my favor, and she was trying to be that hand of support I was going to need. We took the Metro down that day and didn't say much on the ride.

I got to the waiting room and checked in, and looked around as many others were probably waiting for the news that would either put a smile of relief on their face or send their world spinning.

They finally called my name. I tried to muster up a smile as I walked down the hallway and into the examining room. My surgeon walked in. I smiled at him as I tried to read his face. He tried to be as gentle as he could in telling me the news. As I heard the alarming results, 'You have breast cancer,' silence just filled the room. I tried to grasp those words and to be strong as they were whirling around in my head, but finally, letting everything sink in, I just burst into uncontrollable tears.

Funny how no one knows what to say in moments like that. My surgeon just looked on, as he had been in this position many other times. He allowed me to feel what I was feeling at that moment, as the tears running down my face and my body slumped down in the chair told the story of what I was feeling.

Although in my gut I thought that this would be the result, hearing it made it final. After I had gathered myself, I knew that the fight was on. As my doctor tried to ease my mind with what would come next, I tried to put on a brave face. But my mind was doing jumping jacks and somersaults still trying to process the news. I just wanted to leave. He said our next form of action would be a needle biopsy to evaluate the lump felt during my clinical breast exam. He said I could get a second opinion, but I didn't feel it was necessary. I just wanted to move ahead in getting this cancer out of my body.

As we walked back to the Metro, nothing was said. Annie probably felt that I needed silence right now. She was allowing me time to talk when I was ready. Once we got on the Metro, she and I found ourselves laughing at my expression and how I was slumped down in the chair in silence after hearing the results from my surgeon. They say that laughter is good for the soul, and in this case, it was the medicine that I needed. Although I was laughing on the outside, my mind was still busy processing the news. I knew from that moment my life and how I looked at life would be changed forever.

As I sat with my thoughts for the weeks to come, I was trying to pull from everything inspirational I knew to rally myself. I recalled a message I had heard at church years ago. A person had shared a story about her son who was dealing with a circumstance. She had voiced to God that since he had allowed this situation to happen, what was he going to do about it? I turned it around for me and told God that since he had allowed this cancer to come into my body, what was he was going to do about it? I reminded God that I was his responsibility and that he said he would take care of me. I also reminded God of his promise to me that had not come to pass yet, so I knew I couldn't die. I echoed to God that he was a healer and that I was putting the battle of cancer back into his most capable hands. Then I told the Devil that I shall not die.

My surgeon informed me that I would have to have a lumpectomy, which is a partial mastectomy, removing part of the breast tissue. With the lumpectomy, the only removal was the tumor and some surrounding tissue. My surgeon would also remove some of my lymph nodes, which meant I would have to stay in the hospital for a few days.

My surgeon did a second operation on July 1, 1997, a re-excision because the margins weren't clear along, with an axillary node dissection. As they moved me to my room, transferring me to my bed from the gurney, it felt like my arm was ripping from the socket. It was from the incision the surgeon had made in my right armpit to remove some of my lymph nodes to check for cancer cells. I wasn't ready for that heightened pain.

I didn't tell all my family about the breast cancer. For sure not my mom; she was sick, and I didn't need her worrying about me. For the few family members and friends that I did tell, from the start they were worried and afraid. Who wouldn't be when you hear someone has cancer? They concealed their fear and emotions for me. I'm sure when they were alone, they cried for themselves and me because you don't know the overall outcome despite the early diagnoses.

That night I tried my best not to move much, because it meant having to deal with the pain from the cut under my armpit, along with the aftermath of surgery itself. It was hard to turn myself in the bed after surgery because using my chest muscles hurt too much. If I didn't know, I quickly realized their primary function and the anguish I felt using them. The next day, I looked down at my bandaged right breast. As I examined my body, I could see that pinned to my hospital gown was a small drainage tube on my right side. The surgical drain connected to a plastic bulb created suction to help collect excess fluid under my armpit that could accumulate in the area of the tumor. The nurses came in and emptied the fluid from the detachable drain bulb a few times a day into a measuring cup to record the amounts. The drain would be in for a while, even when I left the hospital.

When I left the hospital couple of days later, I was heavily bandaged and only able to move my right arm in a small range of motion. Concealing the plastic bulb bottle to drain fluids was going to be a challenge, knowing how active I was. They filled the implant a little, making my chest area visually uneven on one side. There was now a long scar across the top of my right breast, something that would be present from that point on.

In the days following the lumpectomy, my surgeon would receive a pathology report. This report would explain the characteristics of the breast cancer, and the size of the lump, as well as other diagnostic factors, such as tumor margins and hormone receptor status. This report would help me and my surgeon decide on a treatment plan. When I got out of the hospital, it was over a weekend, so I didn't expect to hear from my surgeon with the results until Monday or Tuesday at the earliest. However, he called me over the weekend. He had gotten the report back early and decided to call me with the results when he said that cancer had not spread and they caught it in the early stages. What a relief. This news was golden, and I didn't have to have chemo. I hung up that phone with my arm raised high and started thanking God.

My treatment would be to undergo adjuvant radiation, the lesser of the two evils. My radiation therapy would be five to seven weeks to eliminate any cancer cells that might still be hiding or present in the remaining breast tissue and to prevent a possible recurrence. Radiation therapy uses a high-energy beam to damage cancer cells. I was diagnosed with ductal carcinoma in situ high-grade with the single focus of microinvasion.

As I prepared for radiation, I had a consultation with the radiation oncologist to review my medical history for treatment and side effects. My next appointment was to get the area marked for treatment. As I laid still for an hour, I watched as they measured and marked my chest with blue ink from my neck down to the area just above my stomach. I thought that my chest was a tic-tac-toe board; the only thing missing was the Xs and O's. They marked and wiped the bleeding blue ink lines drawn across areas of my chest. The radiation oncologist put small marks the size of a pinhead on my skin that would ensure they had correct guides to focus the radiation in the right area for my treatment. The ink lines were temporary, and a few pinpoint permanent marks were also made on my skin.

As they finished and helped me up, I had to digest what I saw on my chest; I looked like something out of a scientific horror movie. As I put on my top, I tried to conceal the blue marking that showed from the upper part of my neck area. I still was trying to hide anything that would give my cancer secret away outside the few people I had told.

Looking in the mirror that night as I removed my clothing, all I saw were blue stains on my shirt and marks covering my entire chest. Not a pretty sight, but a reminder of what was yet to come. Using my right arm was still painful because of the cut under my armpit. The physical therapy gave me exercises to do that would stretch that area out, so that I could get my full range of motion back. One of the exercises was standing in front of a wall and using my fingers to tap up the wall with my arm fully extended. I had to use my left arm to help me get the right arm up the wall because the smarting of the pain was cutting knife-like. When walking, I found myself looking like a stiff board — my right arm looked paralyzed. They told me to just walk naturally with the swinging of my arm. I was trying to figure out the process of doing it since my mind, body, and arm was acting like they were disconnected.

For the next five to seven weeks, the hospital and I were about to become acquainted as I got started with treatment. The radiation treatment only took about 15 minutes, and that was mainly the prep time. When the technicians came to get me, they led me into a room with just a cushioned table in the middle. Above the table was a machine that looked like one of those newspaper or t-shirt presses. Before my treatment started, the radiation team took careful measures to determine the correct angles for aiming the radiation beams and the proper dose of radiation.

As I lay on the table with my right breast exposed, they lined up the machine at the blue marking on my chest. On the outside, I was calm and chatting with the individual getting ready to start the treatment. Inside I was trying to figure out what was about to happen with that piece of machinery that was overshadowing me. As I got ready to have the radiation, it took me back to my days of watching "Star Trek: The Next Generation" and how they could transport someone by a beam of light from the ship to another area. I know that there were beams of light that came down from that machine and zapped me twice. One thing about the treatment, it was not kind to my skin. Gradually, my skin looked like I had sunburn; I never realized how harsh the radiation was. My skin was getting fried like I was in the hot blazing sun with no sun protection on, plus it was itching.

I went for treatment five days per week, and each time it was over, I would head to the gym for a workout. People asked me how I could exercise after getting the radiation. Not knowing any better, I looked at them like they were saying something in a foreign language. Physically it didn't affect me. My stamina and strength were good, despite cancer. I was in good physical condition, which helped with my recovery. Along with the radiation each week, I also had to get my blood drawn just to make sure that my blood levels weren't dropping during treatment.

As life started to get back to normal and after my radiation treatments were over, I made a promise to myself that from that point on I was going to take a vacation to a different destination each year. Having cancer had forced me to look at life a little differently; the time was NOW for me to live. I didn't want to waste any time putting off things.

After finishing all my treatment in 1997, I thought or was hoping that I was finished dealing with cancer. I figured that since the cancer was caught in the earlier stages and I didn't have to undergo chemo, the chances of the cancer returning were slim. How wrong I was! Little did I know cancer was hoisting its ugly head again in my body. In 1998, my mammogram showed no signs of cancer, but throughout the year, I had this acute darting needle-like pain that was shooting through my right breast. My doctors just attributed the pain to the radiation treatment side effects. I didn't argue the matter because although I knew what I felt, there were no signs of cancer, and nothing was showing up that year on my mammogram. Although I was still a little concerned, I tried to put it out of my mind and move on, but the pain would not go away.

I read that life has a way of kicking us when we're down, but just when we think we can't fall any lower, we get kicked again. Unfortunately, it turned out that my 1997 run-in with cancer was not my last. My yearly mammogram in April of 1999 would reveal that cancer had returned, which explained the weight loss I had been experiencing. That news was demoralizing. April was the same month I found out I had cancer in 1997. What a coincidence. Cancer again! I was hoping that my body would not betray me again. I was trying to wrap my head around the thought of having to deal with this again and the unknowing of what this bout of cancer would mean for my life.

I told myself I had done my part after having cancer in 1997. I am a faith walker, and the Bible says in I Corinthians 10:13-14 that God would not put more on you than you can handle, but will always make a way of escape that you can bear. I asked God if he was sure that I could handle this again because I wasn't. That passage of scripture made me question if God knew what he was doing because I did not want to bear this again. How unjustifiable. Why was I facing the ordeal of breast cancer all over again? I questioned if I or the doctor had done anything wrong, or was my initial treatment ineffective?

I read that sometimes microscopic cancer cells, even if it is a single cell, can survive treatment, and they can be too small to be detected. In my research, I had read that rogue cells can remain dormant or continue to multiply, eventually growing until they are large enough to be felt or found on a mammogram. I figured this was what happened in my case, because in 1998, nothing showed up on the mammogram even though I had these darting pains in my right breast.

This second fight with cancer would prove to be a little more challenging than the first time. The cancer was close to my chest wall. Fortunately, once again it didn't break outside my chest wall and spread throughout my body. This was an enormous challenge for me as a woman, as it would be for any woman. This time I was losing my right breast and enduring so much more. No woman wants to lose her breast. My surgeon had informed me the first time that if the cancer did return, the breast would have to go because you cannot give radiation therapy to the same area twice. However, when looking at the bigger picture, choosing life versus the breast removal is a no-brainer. I was thinking, was I supposed to learn something that I hadn't the first time around?

By not knowing all the details about cancer in my body this time around, I felt like my mom and all my siblings needed to know. There would be a lot more that would go into my surgery and recovery this time around so I would need all hands on deck. I honestly had to stand on the promises of God again and his word, because God's word was the only reliable thing I knew could help me stay steadfast when my world was spinning what felt like out of control. At this point for me, it was once again about getting this cancer out of my body and about my emotional and psychological adjustments. My mind and emotions were in a war at that moment. I was fighting with my emotions to accept once again what I had to face.

As I prepared for my doctor's visit, my former surgeon retired. Having a new doctor was the least of my real concerns, because the person taking over for him was one of the best from my research. My breast surgeon this time around was a female who had taken over for my former surgeon.

The first procedure was an excisional biopsy on April 26, 1999, which they did with wire localization. Once again it would be done in the ambulatory building across from the hospital. Doing the procedure, it felt like they were jamming that machine through my chest. The cancer was close to my chest wall in the lower quadrant; therefore, they had to make sure that they got the margins and marking right. My face was an imprint in the plastic glass of the machine by being so close to it. By the time they finished, I felt like the machine and I were the same. Had the tech pushed my chest forward anymore, my chest was going to go right through the machine. Once the results were back, I met with my surgeon to talk about the mastectomy.

My sister Nettie and a few close friends went with me for my appointment to discuss my options. As we waited for the surgeon to come in, we all tried to put on a good face, but looking at them I felt their nervousness as I felt my own.

When the doctor came in, she tried her best to help me understand the procedure and prepare me psychologically. I sat there looking at her as she explained the options in removing my breast. She said that I could choose not to have reconstruction and have it flat and use a breast prosthesis. A breast prosthesis made with silicone gel or another material would fit either on my chest or directly in the pocket of a particular bra. Another option was to delay reconstruction, and the third was to do it immediately following the mastectomy operation to remove my breast and then insert the expander for the implant. When I heard "Do nothing and leave it flat," I missed everything else she said, my ears went deaf. I began to tear up and almost started crying. It was becoming a little overwhelming and my bravery showed some cracks in the armor.

The words rushed out of my mouth so fast: "No, I can't have it flat." As I calmed myself down, Nettie and my friends reassured me that it would be all right. I decided to go with the immediate reconstruction after the mastectomy. That way I didn't have to have another surgery later. Although there were two more options, I wasn't a candidate for either. Before my mastectomy, I met with the reconstruction doctor that would be doing the injections to the expander.

It's surgery day, June 1, 1999, and one of my most endearing parts will be gone, my right breast. So much was going on that day to prepare me for surgery I didn't have time to cry or be emotional about it.

The mastectomy surgery took two to three hours because I was also getting reconstruction performed at the same time. As I awakened from surgery, I looked down at my chest to examine it; it was wrapped from one end to the other with bandages. My breasts were not as they had once been. One side was higher and the other side appeared to be deflated. The bandages empowered me to deal with the reality of my right breast being gone. It was challenging moving around in the bed. It was painful because every muscle in my chest was throwing jab punches at me. Pinned to my gown this time were two drainage bottles. They would be with me for a few weeks until all the fluids drained. I was in the hospital for three days.

When my family came to visit me, we all tried to keep everything upbeat. I think we all just wanted to move from cancer and the surgery to recovery. I know I did. As I prepared to go home, I allowed myself the time to feel whatever I needed to feel for me to move forward.

However, I still didn't want to spend a lot of time being upset or in a dark place. It was vital for me to get back to living.

Although they had put in the tissue expander, it would be months before the implant could go in. For now, I had to deal with the flatness of my breast. What the tissue expander would do was stretch my remaining chest skin and soft tissue to make room for the breast implant. My surgeon placed a balloon-like tissue expander under my pectoral muscle at the time of my mastectomy. Over the next months, through a small valve under my skin, my plastic surgeon would use a needle to inject saline into the valve, filling the balloon in stages. The more they filled it, I experienced some discomfort as the pressure started to build and the implant expanded, it felt like the expander was going to pop, it was so tight. It looked like I had a mini bowling ball on my chest.

Not long after the surgery, my mom came to Maryland for a visit. One day while we were sitting around, I told her about having cancer this time and why I didn't tell her about my first bout with breast cancer. I informed her that she was sick. I acknowledged that I didn't want her worrying, that my concern was more for her and what she was going through. She understood.

From the outside, with clothing on, no one would have guessed anything was different with me. I decided to hold off having the nipple and areola reconstruction. The procedure included tattooing to define the dark area of skin surrounding my nipple. I was more focused on allowing my new breast time to heal along with my overall self.

In the upcoming weeks and months, my plastic surgeon would inject through a tiny valve under my skin a salt-water solution at regular intervals to fill the expander. She did this over a period of four to six months. By the end of those six months, my pumped-up right breast was so tight and hard that if I had bumped into anyone they would have thought they were running into a brick wall. After the skin over the breast area has stretched enough, I had to go back in for a second surgery to remove the expander and put in the permanent implant. Cosmetically, the look wasn't what I had before, but at least I had something there that I could play off with clothing.

In months down the road, the teardrop implant they had put in to feel like my natural breast had flipped. I noticed that the implant was almost up in my neck area. The bottom was now at the top. They removed that implant and replaced it with a round shape. Although this one was still not a perfect fit, I just decided to deal with what I had because I was tired of all the surgeries.

My doctors wanted me to begin taking the prescription drug Tamoxifen, which is used to treat breast cancer patients. Tamoxifen citrate had been the most commonly prescribed drug to treat breast cancer since the approval of the drug by the U.S. Food and Drug Administration (FDA) in the 1970s. I decided to bypass this drug because, in reading up on it, it had too many side effects. I felt those side effects outweighed the purpose of the drug. I also told the doctor that I didn't want the hormone therapy. I just wanted to move forward, and having to deal with the side effects of this drug would not have kept my mind at ease.

I told my doctor that I was going to believe God for my total healing. I was entrusting my life into God's most capable hands and believing his word in Isaiah 53:5, which stated that "He was wounded for our transgressions, He was bruised for our iniquities; The chastisement for our peace was upon Him, and by His stripes, we are healed." One of the other main reasons I didn't want to take Tamoxifen was because if I wanted to have children, I would have to wait five years, and being already in my mid-30s, I didn't want that window to close. My doctor said that in five years or so there would be other drugs coming out that might be better than Tamoxifen, so I decided that the choice I made was the best one for me. At the time, it was all about taking the time to heal and not worrying about something else that might affect my body.

In anything that you go through in life, I believe that you can always turn a negative into a positive. One day, I was talking to Hall of Famer and former NFL cornerback Darrell Green after my second bout with breast cancer. As a sports broadcaster, I had covered the Washington Redskins for most of his career. He and I had become friends, more like family. I felt a pull from God to do something with what I had gone through, and I was discussing this with him.

Sometimes when you go through adversity, you don't know how God is cultivating what you went through, to put purpose and meaning in it, not just for you but others.

Being in sports for most of my life, and playing basketball for so many years before college and after, Darrell said I should start a basketball tournament to raise money for breast cancer survivors in the Washington metropolitan area. He said, "Don't reinvent the wheel, but do what you know." I started a basketball fundraiser for young and older adults in 2000. I joined the Breast Cancer Care Foundation, an organization started by my breast surgeon and other individuals I met during my treatment. They had the same vision as I did, so it was a perfect fit, and they welcomed me. I donated all the money raised from my tournament to the foundation. I told myself I would stay under their umbrella and learn all the details about starting and running a charity. I gave myself five years, and after that, I would start my foundation, Hopkins Breast Cancer Inc., the helping hand in the community, a charity that meets the immediate needs of individuals surviving breast cancer in the Washington metropolitan area.

Life is so precious and not guaranteed, nor are our conditions. When thinking about life's path, it will not always be paved with a smooth surface, and it will not always reveal the dark moments that await us. No, I didn't like the fact that cancer came into my body not once but twice.

It is hard to thank God for the tough times in our lives, but when we can, we are made so much stronger. My journey through two bouts of breast cancer was a walk of faith and trust. I often tell people that I took a few hits for the kingdom, so I could stand in the gap for someone else who might have to go through the same thing. My will to live was stronger than cancer that engulfed my body both times.

I was at one of my doctor's appointments when my doctor stepped out of the room for a minute. I glanced at my big fat medical chart before she returned to examine me. Inside she noted, "Great attitude, good spirit, always upbeat with a smile on her face." She believed these were elements that helped in my healing. What she did not realize was there was a fight that God had placed in me long before the cancer entered my body.

The scientific community won't admit it, but I believe they have seen enough cases to know that those with a positive attitude have a better outcome, along with those who have their faith and belief in God. I was at a scientific meeting, and they asked about me being a breast cancer survivor, but more notably, they wanted to know about my relationship with my doctors after my diagnosis and my cure from cancer and years after. Being a cancer patient, it's not like it's a quick fix; it's more of a journey, a roadmap to the unknowing. It may start off as doctor and patient, but it soon becomes a bonding connection, almost like a mother feeling the kick of her unborn child and understanding what each kick means.

My current breast doctor said that she sees the first encounter as crisis prevention, letting the person know that although it is terrible what you are going through, you the patient are going to come out at the end and be okay. I especially like what she said in our closing conversation, that relationships in crisis are forged. I want to say cultivated. In going through cancer twice, it made me understand how vital the doctor and a patient relationship has to be. There must be trust on both sides.

In 2017, in my search to find out the stage of my cancer, I uncovered something that I wasn't prepared to hear from my breast doctor: that I had aggressive breast cancer. I had this perplexed look on my face like she must be mistaken. As I questioned her more, my voice had this concerned tone, and my mind was in overdrive. She said in 1999, she stated that the surgical pathology diagnosis reading showed that I had infiltrating ductal carcinoma, 0.3 cm, poorly differentiated (grade III of III) meaning on the aggressive side, triple negative, which was aggressive breast cancer. She did point out that it was only 0.3 cm small, and it was detected early. I felt somewhat better, but the voice in my ear was still echoing that I had aggressive breast cancer.

Part of me was glad that I didn't know it in 1997 and 1999. I asked her did most people get aggressive breast cancer, she said only 15 percent did, and more African-American women did. It was not something my ears wanted to hear, but useful information. As I left her office, I couldn't shake the feeling of hearing about having aggressive breast cancer.

Yes, cancer took hold of my body twice and had a brief stay, but in the process of going through it all, I refused to allow it to be the winner in my soul and the regulator and dimmer of my spirit. Years later, as I think about each bout with breast cancer, some of the details of the procedures and treatments have faded, but what is crystal clear that comes flooding back from time to time is all of the emotions that I felt throughout the process of dealing with the disease. You can see the effects of cancer which are seen by the scars on the surface of my body, they are part of my story, but they do not define who I am. In fact, they tell me that I am a survivor, a fighter, a warrior, an overcomer with a winning attitude to move forward to victory.

We might never understand why things happen as they do, or come against us, or why we might have to go through the same thing again and again; but one thing we can always count on is that we have someone who will always stand in the gap and fight for us. God assures us in many ways that he has never entered a fight where he has not come out the winner in the end. In Jeremiah 30:17 it states God "will restore you to health and heal your wounds, declares the LORD."

4
MY LAST WALK FOR A MINUTE

────◄ ◆ ● ◆ ►────

*True strength is when you have a lot to cry about, but you
choose to smile and take another step forward instead.*
— C. TANG

walked to the hospital that warm summer day without
a care in the world, music blasting in my ears, never
thinking or even imagining how my life would soon
be altered in the most unforeseeable way. I was about to
get hit by a metaphorical freight train that I didn't even see
coming my way. There were no warning signs; no one was
there yelling for me to get off the tracks. Before I knew it,
I was hit.

My present walk would be a life-changing misfortune.

On June 2, 2010, I was on the phone with Dr. A's office.
They said my surgery to remove uterus fibroid tumors
would be at 3 p.m., not my ideal time. I don't like having

surgery that late in the day, not that I love having it at all. I prefer to be the first person in the morning, while everyone is fresh and energetic.

They wanted me to arrive at noon on June 3, to do a blood test before surgery, making sure that my blood levels were okay. I asked if I was going to need blood for surgery; they said no. I had my sister Nettie on standby just in case. She had that golden blood, the O negative which she could give to all blood types. I asked how long I was going to be in the hospital. They confirmed what I was thinking — five days at most.

In an email, my friend Cindy asked about my surgery, confirming the date. I told her and conveyed that Annie, another friend, was going to bring my bag over after surgery since I planned on walking over to the hospital.

In my email conversation with Cindy, I stated that it would be my last good walk for a minute. I told her to notice I said; "for a minute." She wrote back, "Your body is healthy, so you are right, a minute!" Amazing how haunting that email would be later.

For years, I had uterus fibroid tumors, noticed first during a yearly gynecologist appointment at one of the local hospitals. At that time, they were the size of a dime, but over the years several had grown to the size of softballs. With all my previous surgeries, a right ACL knee injury, breast cancer twice, and thyroid Graves' disease, I loathed having any surgery.

Regardless of wanting to shrug at another surgery, it was a necessity because the uterine fibroid tumors were causing chronic bleeding and putting extra pressure on my bladder, which made me feel like I always had to go to the bathroom. My current GYN physician did an ultrasound, among other tests, and determined that I was nowhere close to menopause. He suggested having a hysterectomy, which would eliminate the tumors.

My doctor had given me the name of one of the top gynecologic oncologists in the area, Dr. A. I met with him to go over my options and decided, as my GYN had suggested, on having the hysterectomy. However, after thinking about it weeks before my surgery, I decided to have just the fibroid tumors removed since I still wanted to keep the door open for having children.

Although I might have been a little late in life to be even thinking about this, I wanted that option. Besides, nothing was wrong with my uterus, so I felt no need to go the hysterectomy route. I informed Dr. A of the change, and his office sent new paperwork.

Dr. A had discussed with me the laparoscope option, which is a surgical procedure in which a fiber-optic instrument is inserted through the abdominal wall to view the organs, and either remove the fibroids or block blood flow to the fibroids.

I wish that I had read up a little more on the risk factors to know more about some of the more severe complications of the laparoscopy. Some of the risks are damage to an abdominal blood vessel, the bladder, the bowel, the uterus, and other pelvic structures; nerve damage; allergic reactions; blood clots; and problems with urinating.

The year of 2010 was going to be a busy and eventful year for me, my friends and my family. My nephew in West Virginia was graduating high school in early May and my niece was graduating high school in Maryland in June. I was also going to Greece on vacation in July with some of my family and friends. I was embarking upon the big 5-0, so I was treating myself to an early birthday present with the trip. In fact, I was going to plan a lot of things leading up to my birthday month in November but, during those arrangements, I had to schedule a surgery around everything.

On my surgery day, I decided to go to work for a few hours in the morning. Once I got back home, I packed a bag and left it for Annie before heading over to the hospital. As I headed out in my flip flops, a skirt, and a colorful light green top, I put on my headphones to listen to music on the walk over. Never did I think that I wouldn't be walking out the same way I walked in. My world was about to change in a way that I never saw coming. I was about to be blindsided, my life was going to be stricken, and the damage would be quite injurious.

They were admitting me to the hospital for elective myomectomy of uterine fibroids that were causing chronic bleeding. As I sat there waiting to complete paperwork, I still had my headphones on, listening to music and looking around, studying everyone coming and going. As I waited, I wasn't thinking about much, not even the surgery itself, since I had done this so many times before. Anything going wrong didn't enter my mind.

My family and a few friends arrived at the hospital after my surgery was over. Dr. A informed them that everything had gone well. They had removed 13 fibroid tumors, using a diagnostic laparoscopy, exploratory laparotomy and abdominal myomectomy of the fibroids. There were no complications and estimated blood loss was a liter. However, later that night, Dr. A came in before my family left and was concerned that the catheter to drain urine from my bladder was filling up with blood.

On Friday, June 4, day two, Annie called my family to let them know Dr. A and Dr. B were taking me back into surgery. They thought I was bleeding internally since the bottle was continually filling up with blood. I had a two-unit blood transfusion. They informed my family that I was hemodynamically stable, meaning my blood flow was now stable and the blood circulation was good. So, rather than delay the surgery until I was unstable, both doctors had elected to return to the operating room for exploration and evaluation. There was approximately 300 mL of dark blood in my pelvis, which was a substantial loss of blood. So that the doctors could remove the 300 mL of dark blood, a drain was placed in my abdomen and pelvis. However, there was no active bleeding identified. After somewhat of a scare, there was no complication, and on day three, Saturday, June 5, I was doing great. In fact, I was up walking around, but before I could be released, I had to have a bowel movement.

On Sunday, June 6, to my surprise, I had a room full of visitors: friends, family, and people from my church, along with my pastor. I was somewhat tired and told my family that there were too many people in the room.

My sister Nettie and Cindy looked at each other like, "who's going to be the bad cop?" They told my visitors that it was entirely too tiring for me and had most individuals leave so that I could get some rest. After that, they limited who would come and told everyone that I was not up for visitors, but to please keep me in their prayers. Although I was thankful that people cared enough to visit, I found out that it is so important to monitor visitors early on, because I just had two surgeries within three days of being in the hospital. My body was still in the initial stages of healing so it might have been just a little too early for all those visitors. Even though I looked all right, my body was still fighting off whatever was still happening inside.

On day five of my hospital stay, everything was still going well. In fact, they were thinking about letting me out. However, I caught an infection over the weekend, which they dealt with right away. My mom was in town for my niece Nettiel's graduation, and I knew she felt better once she saw me for herself. I kept telling her on the phone, "I'm okay, mother, I'm a soldier," and I told her to just take care of herself.

For whatever reason, on Tuesday I started feeling sick. My brother-in-law's mother, who had also come in for Nettiel's graduation wanted to see me, but they told her that she needed to wait because I wasn't feeling well.

That Wednesday, June 9, day seven, I started to feel sick. I was complaining about feeling nauseous and when I used the bathroom my lower intestines weren't working, but the upper ones were. I was also feeling tired. Earlier that day, a couple of friends dropped by for a visit, but I told them I wasn't feeling very well and could barely keep my eyes open while they were there, so they left.

The doctors decided to put a tube down my nose to look at my stomach. The nurses told my family, "This is not the Donna we knew from a day or so ago. She is not her usual upbeat self."

The male nurse came back into my room and told my sister Nettie and friend Cindy that they had to put on gowns and masks. They were sitting on the couch in my room, and both looked at each other trying to figure out what was going on. Later the doctor came in and said I had an infection. That was the start of my health's downhill spiral.

My family was the only visitors allowed because of the bacterial infection and when they came into my room, they had to wear gowns, masks, and gloves.

I turned off my cellphone and the hospital phones because they were ringing and beeping too much. Plus, I still had the tube in my nose and would have to keep it in for another day. Therefore, it was difficult for me to talk anyway. Finally, after much prayer, I was passing gas, and they said I was on the mend.

My medical records noted that I experienced several bouts of nausea and vomiting, along with not having a return of bowel movements or flatus, which were further signs of an intestinal abnormality. I was under observation for a distended abdomen; the doctors suspected ileus, which is a lack of movement somewhere in my intestines. Ileus is a blockage of food material, gas, and liquids that could not get through. The distention of my abdomen worsened that day and was described as "tympanic to percussion," likening my abdominal muscles to the tightly drawn membrane of a drum. Also during this time, I was diagnosed with Clostridium difficile colitis, bacteria that caused swelling and irritation of my large intestine and colon. Additionally, I was having problems with my blood chemistry, low levels of calcium, and kidney function.

Before June 10, my blood laboratory work reflected continuing anemia, with platelet counts that were within normal limits. I thought that I was on the mend, but on the morning of June 10, day eight, I reported a new complaint of "numbness to the plantar surface" of my left foot. I was still able to get out of bed and walk around the hospital, but the medical report further noted that I exhibited a good range of motion in my left foot and my calves were not tender. I had no abnormal swelling in my legs or feet. However, I still wasn't getting any better, so they moved me to the critical care unit (CCU) where they could monitor me better. The nurses were glad that I was transferred to the CCU.

A physical therapy consultation was ordered to address my left foot paresthesia, which felt like something was crawling on my skin. My foot was tingling, numb, and itching. That afternoon, Dr. B had me transferred to the intensive care unit (ICU), under his care. This was following episodes of an increasingly rapid heart rate in addition to my worsening abdominal distention and kidney problems, which had progressed to a condition of systemic inflammatory response syndrome. A grave situation was arising from my body's immune response to the infection associated with a potential for organ failure. At this point, there was a significant concern by both Dr. B and Dr. C surrounding my intestine. The evening of June 10, I was taken back to the operating room by Doctors B and C, who recommended surgical re-exploration of my abdomen. They said that they were going to do surgery to see if I had a blockage in my upper bowels or intestines because my stomach was hard, and my heart was racing, plus I had a fever. Since my first surgery on June 3, this was my third surgery.

Dr. C and A took me back to surgery for another procedure, the procedure was an exploratory laparotomy for lysis of adhesions, resulted in a total abdominal hysterectomy. They surveyed the entire length of my intestine and colon but could not identify the location of any obstructions;

they further found no signs of intra-abdominal abscess or bowel compromise.

There was a significant amount of clear fluid found in my abdomen, which was consistent with the inflammatory response. When the fluid was cultured, tests reviewed systemic inflammatory response syndrome with sepsis, with a possible abdominal source. Dr. A did a hysterectomy, removing my uterus to ensure that it wasn't the source of my infection. It wasn't, and it had nothing to do with the issues I was having. Although the first surgery went well, pathologic analysis of my uterus revealed some surgical trauma of the myomectomy surgery to remove the fibroids. Still, this wasn't why my body was in distress at this point.

Dr. A wanted to remove my uterus when he did the surgery for the fibroid tumors, but I had requested that he leave my uterus because I tried to keep the door open for having children. However, it had to be removed anyway after surgery number three due to my ongoing health issues. Dr. A was still puzzled after that third surgery because they didn't find any reason why I was still having problems. The other doctors assigned to my case who were checking on the blockage said they found nothing and would continue to treat my infection. I remained under the care of the critical care specialists following my June 10 surgery.

On June 11, I told my niece Alisha, who was going to stay with me at the hospital, that my foot felt like it was falling asleep. I had pressure cuffs on my legs since my first surgery. Alisha told the nurse and doctors the concern I had with my foot falling asleep. She would periodically rub my foot, and the feeling and color would come back.

Later that evening, my abdominal distention had worsened, and I complained to the staff of tenderness at the site of the third surgical incision. My legs were also noticeably swollen, which was raising concerns among the hospital staff of the possibility of compartment syndrome. Compartment syndrome is a condition in which increased intramuscular pressure brought about by swelling and edema becomes high enough to impair blood flow; this was critical because compartment syndrome is potentially very dangerous. It can result in nerve damage and the need for amputation of the affected limbs.

The next morning, Saturday, June 12, I still had a tube in 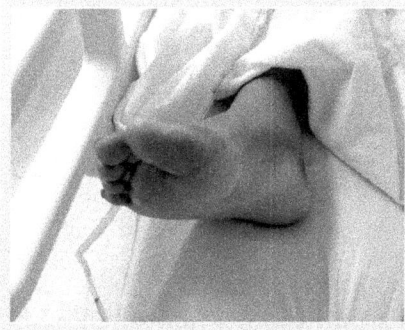 my nose, and I again complained about my arm and leg being numb. My sister Nettie arrived at the hospital during the early morning before taking her two daughters to dance rehearsal. I had the hospital blankets off my feet, and she noticed my left foot looked purple.

She asked my niece Alisha and sister Carolyn if they had seen it, which they hadn't. Alisha told her about me complaining about my foot falling asleep and being numb. Nettie went to the nurse and asked him if he had noticed that my toes were purple. He said no and came to look at them. He said my foot was not like that the last time he checked and said he would have someone look at it.

My left arm was tense with swelling, and my left leg was numb and discol-ored, which the doctors described as mildly duskier than the right leg. Both legs were cool to the touch, indi-cating a degree of impairment to the flow of blood to both legs.

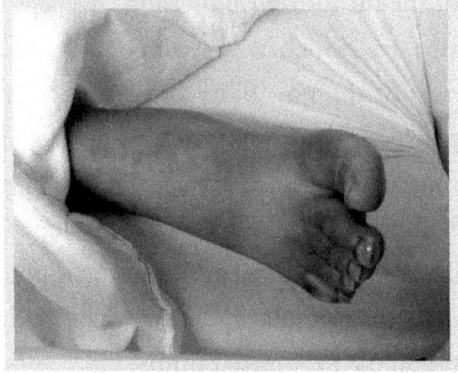

Throughout the day, I wasn't getting better, and in fact, I was getting worse. My body was retaining fluid and I was swollen. My blood pressure and heart rate were high. I had a fever, was in pain, and was having trouble breathing. I was in renal failure, and my kidneys were functioning only minimally. No one at this point could figure out why my body was in elevated distress.

Because of the problem with my left foot and leg, they did a Doppler ultrasound test, which is used to measure the amount of blood flow through your arteries and veins that supply blood to your arms and legs. They were lis-tening for a pulse. In the meantime, Nettie called Cindy. When Cindy arrived, she was alarmed upon seeing my foot.

Nettie informed her that she had already pointed this out to the nurse. One of the nurses told my family that I was not doing well. He said by the time patients get to him; they should be 24 to 48 hours from being released from the hospital. His remarks indicated that I seemed to be regressing.

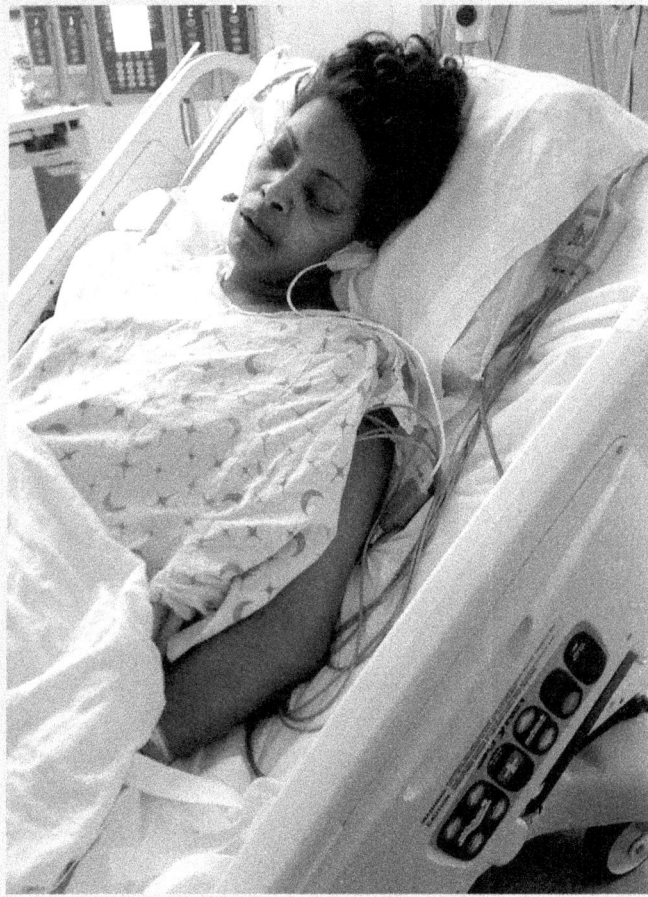

At this point, my condition kept deteriorating. Both Nettie and Cindy were sitting in those yellow gowns huddled together, wondering what in the world was going on. Later that morning an order for Heparin was placed on my chart, and I was given a dose of the anti-coagulation medication. But soon after, the Heparin was discontinued, and an evaluation was ordered to investigate whether I might have an adverse response to Heparin.

At midday on June 12, Dr. A noted in my chart that I had generalized swelling throughout my body, such that the pulses of my femoral arteries could not be felt in either one of my legs. My left leg appeared slightly dusky with a sluggish capillary refill, meaning that when Dr. A pressed his finger into my swollen leg, the area he touched remained pale for slightly longer than he considered normal.

Within ten days, I had had three surgeries. By now I thought that I would have been at home recovering, but instead, my body was in extreme distress, and no one could figure out why. The doctors were baffled.

> Cindy: *One day I was there from about 6:30 p.m. until 12:30 a.m. Donna's skin color was a little off. Her mom, Alisha and Nettie came by and stayed for a while, then left. Annie had gotten there for the night shift at 12:30 a.m.; she said it was a long night. Around 2 a.m., she stated that Donna's heart was racing, even though she wasn't feeling it, so they did an EKG, and it came out okay.*

I was being fed through a tube still, and my condition was worsening. At this point, the doctors sounded the alarms.

Dr. A, the critical care physician, and the vascular surgeon were in consultation concerning the condition of my left leg and the recommendation at this point. The vascular surgeon recommended having me brought to the operating room as soon as possible for surgical treatment of compartment syndrome. At this stage I was so sick, I was not aware of anything that was going on around me. My signature on the surgery consent form looked like chicken scratch.

On June 12, they performed a fasciotomy by cutting the skin on my left leg, which allowed the compartments to expand, which reduced the intra-compartmental pressures to restore blood flow. In my case, a four-venogram test of my veins to let them see 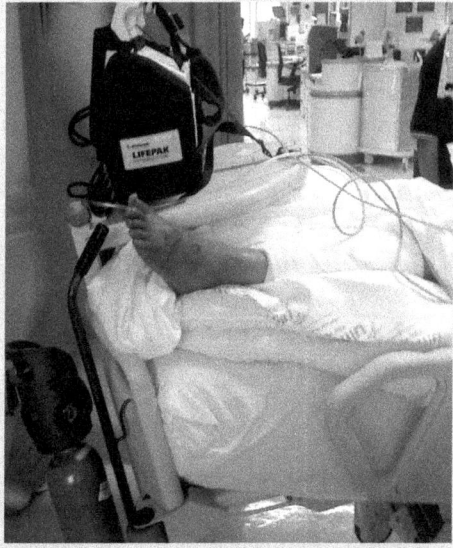 the blood vessels in my left leg showed good blood flow through the arteries down through my mid-calf. There was a weaker flow when it got to my foot, but no identifiable embolic or thrombotic lesions.

On Sunday, June 13, day 11, my foot color was still not improving, and my other health issues were still not good.

I was still complaining of pain and numbness in my left leg and foot. At 8:07 a.m., a doctor who was a second-year surgical resident wrote in my chart that there continued to be no palpable or Dopplerable signal of the left lower extremity since my June 12 surgery, meaning that adequate blood flow to my left foot had not returned despite the fasciotomy. She further remarked that she anticipated the health care providers would wait for a signal that the blood flow returning to the foot had allowed tissue to detach, which meant that amputation would be inevitable.

Cindy: *I was directed to take my oil and anoint and pray for Donna. I had left the house on the way to the hospital and turned back because I had forgotten the oil. Bob, my husband, said, "You got your oil? " I said yes. He told me to be careful with that in the hospital. All I knew is what God had directed me to do. This time I knew, I knew what was up, the foot began to turn purple again. I asked Donna, "Is there anything too hard for God?" She shook her head no. I anointed her from top to bottom, arms, legs, stomach, everything. I told her we would fight it, all of it.*

They were taking Donna in and out of her room so much from one surgery to the next, that Nettie, Alisha,

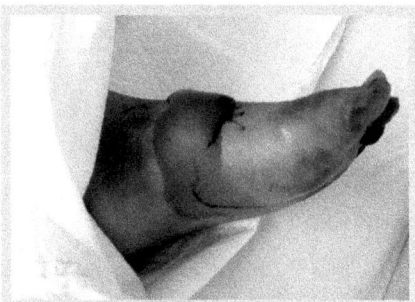

and I were all running behind her bed frantically when they were wheeling her toward pre-op. By the fourth surgery, they were trying to see if they could transfer Donna elsewhere because it was apparent they didn't have a clue what was going on.

By the fourth surgery, Donna was a bit delirious, in and out of lucidity, she was holding something in her hands (it may have been her iPod) and praying, and that's when Alisha was sitting in my lap. We began to pray too. Nettie was talking to a friend of the family whose brother was a doctor at a hospital in Boston, and they were gathering his thoughts about what should be done. He talked to the nurse who was on duty, and from that conversation, he gave us information about what was going on and it wasn't good.

Marcy: *I was naturally worried from the start about Donna going in for surgery, even though she was upbeat the day of the first surgery at the first hospital. I remember her saying that she was going to walk to the hospital from her house. After surgery, I checked in on her, and she told me she was doing fine. She was telling me that she had even walked around the floor.*

Perhaps that erased my skepticism or more than likely I sounded skeptical. To prove she was doing well, Donna sent a picture of herself sitting up in bed laughing and looking great! I must say, I never rested until she was home safely.

I hadn't arrived yet, but when things started going wrong, I was receiving detailed, blow- by-blow texts as Donna's health deteriorated, and it was happening so fast it was gut-wrenching. I remember someone telling me that a black male nurse was very concerned, saying this isn't the vibrant woman who came in and is not the person she was a day or so ago. He seemed to say something was terribly wrong, sounding a warning.

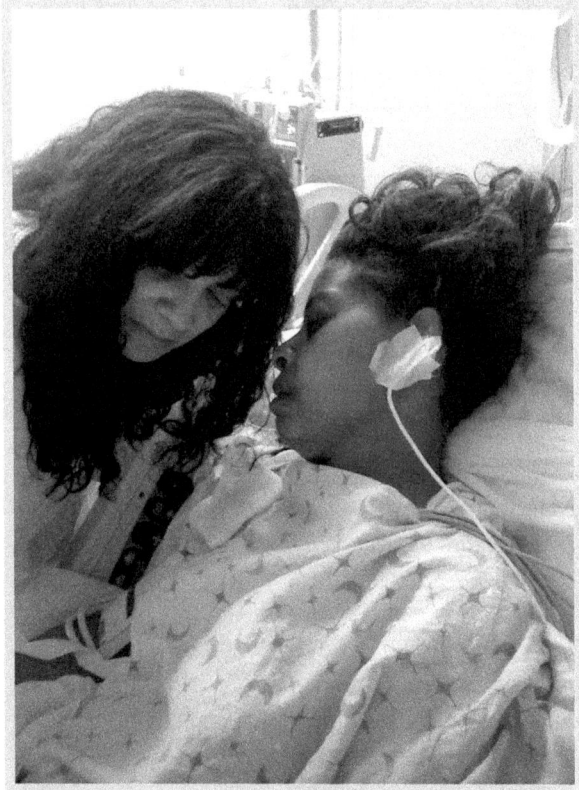

I distinctly remember the day I arrived. Donna was in the ICU at the first hospital. By then she had started to swell throughout her body. She was aware I was there, but I am not sure how much registered. Donna had a song playing on a continuous loop — it was either "I Speak Life," or "I Shall Not Die," or something like that. I'm not even sure if she remembers the title. As the evening and night wore on, Donna would panic as the recording stopped and wanted it turned back on immediately.

She was dozing in and out of sleep. When Donna did wake up, she was asking for ice. At this point, she started to become disoriented and delusional and finished the whole cup. She would automatically do the breathing exercises to keep her lungs clear and then doze back off, wake up, ask for ice, eat it all, do breathing exercises, and doze back off again.

This pattern continued all through the night. For urine monitoring purposes, the hospital staff would only give me ice for her in one small Styrofoam cup at a time. I remember the nurses getting aggravated because of my repeated requests for ice.

I remember seeing Donna's toes turning purple and alerted the nurse, then watching the purple progress up the foot. Healthy pink areas would become white, then purple. The staff used a marker to draw a horizontal line across the bottom of her foot to determine if the lack of circulation was progressing and it continued to move past each mark. The leg and foot — Donna's whole body still

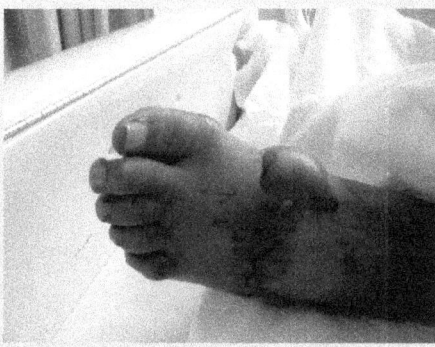

had significant swelling. I remember watching Donna's urine bag and the urine getting darker. It was like so many things were going wrong at the same time, and no one had answers. The medical staff seemed to have more and more questions they couldn't answer or solve. Donna continued to be non-coherent. It was like she understood questions and could answer them. She would complain about her symptoms but clearly was not herself mentally.

Then she began complaining about her hand and arm being numb or bothering her, and we could see a slight change in the color, turning white then a blue tinge. We all were scared because she had so much swelling, the initial diagnosis was a result of capsular contraction, indicating that the fluid-filled tissue was applying too much pressure to the veins and arteries and basically cutting off circulation. That's why they performed the first operation on the leg, to open it up and relieve the pressure.

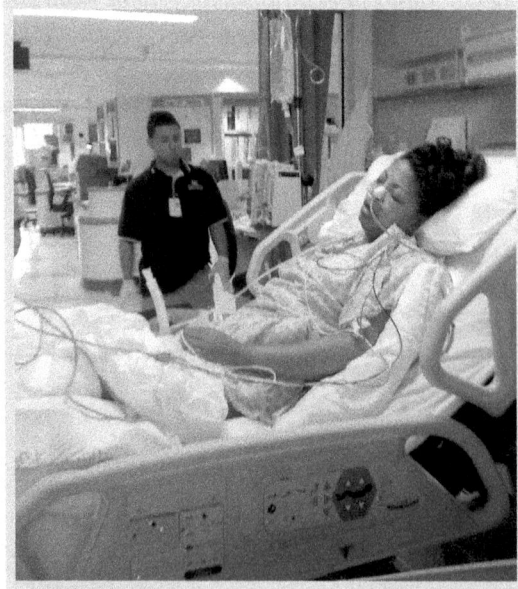

That didn't work, and the purple movement continued, and now the first areas turned purple and then black. My

heart sunk! I knew that once the tissue turned black, it could never be saved. And they still had no clue what was happening. It was evident they were in over their heads.

Donna had continued to complain of the same issues with her hands and shoulder and arm, so they took her down to determine if she had blood clots in those areas. They brought her back up and said they had broken up clots found in her upper body. I was only at the first hospital for two days, and it felt like two weeks. Thinking back on it, from the time I arrived in her room that Saturday, Donna was wheeled out of her room for four procedures, three of which were surgical. It was gut-wrenching not knowing if she would come back up, and happy when she did, only to face the fact that she was continuing to decline at a rapid rate and no medical professional had a clue what was going on.

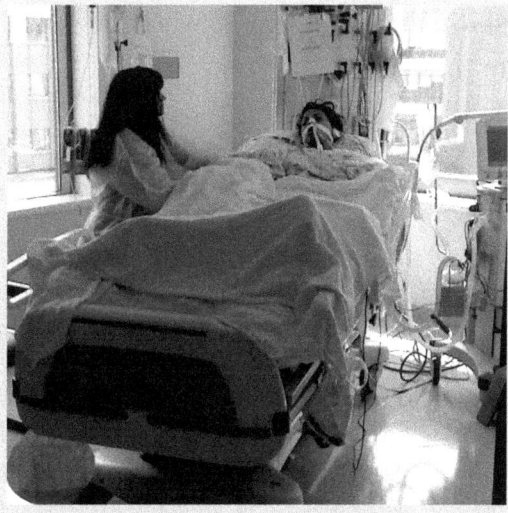

Early one morning a young resident came in, he was fresh out of medical school; I was so desperate I began explaining symptoms to him looking for answers from

anywhere. He thought for a bit, and you could see the light bulb go off in his head: HIT, heparin-induced thrombocytopenia. No one had even thought of that.

My other health issues weren't getting any better. I was still having trouble breathing, my kidneys were only functioning at a small percentage, and my blood pressure and heart rate were still up, among other problems. Later that evening, my doctors, along with a senior consultant level doctor, decided that serious consideration should be given to transferring me to a tertiary care center, a hospital that has personnel and facilities for advanced medical investigation, which provides health care from specialists in a more substantial hospital. At this point, I wanted to be moved to another hospital, so when they asked me if I wanted to go, I said yes.

Cindy: *The hospital said that what Donna was going through was outside of their capabilities, and they were transferring her to the second hospital, which was in Baltimore. They told me she was stable enough to be transported by ambulance. Everyone had gone home because they said it would be between 10:15 p.m. and 7 a.m. Her sister Carolyn called and told Nettie they planned to transfer her in the next two hours, and Nettie, Carolyn and I followed the ambulance down, driving like crazy to keep up with the ambulance. Nettie had on her four-way flashers and went through every stop sign or red light the ambulance went through. I told Nettie not to let that ambulance out of our sight! At one point, we were doing 90-95 mph. We got to Baltimore about 1 a.m., and they started from scratch evaluating Donna that night.*

As morning came on Monday June 14, Nettie and I were planning to go home and get ready for work, albeit late. Just as we were about to leave Donna with Carolyn, a female surgeon came out at about 5 a.m. and said, "We have to take her into surgery." Honestly, at first, I don't think I processed what she said. She said, "We have to relieve the pressure on that leg." Admittedly, it was looking bad, like you could pop it with a needle. Nettie was in shock and folded over in half, I dropped to the chair and was just shaking my head, I think. They were trying to save Donna's foot and had bumped other surgeries to get her in quickly. Nettie had to sign the papers because at this time Donna was so drugged.

Nettie looked at me mystified because the surgeon was telling her the possible outcome: gangrene, death, amputation. I said, "Nettie, we do what we must do to save her life," but I refused to allow the enemy to take her foot. I know Donna didn't have any idea where she was. They did the surgery and left Donna's leg open. I must say despite what was going on; it was awesome to see—her veins and muscles were perfect, like in one of those science books.

At this point, they had saved the foot. They had a pulse before Nettie, and I left. Marcy said Donna pointed to her foot with the question in her eyes and Marcy said she and Annie told her that her foot was okay and to rest. She told me you could see the relief and tears in Donna's eyes.

The top portion of the foot is black and deteriorating, especially the big toe and the one beside it.

This female surgeon at the Medical Center, she is harsh and direct, she doesn't mince words, but she is real and honest. She met with the family; we were all on overload. Her mom was there with her Aunt Eloise. Donna's Aunt Eloise had her rosary beads, and she was rolling them fast. The female surgeon told the family that they would have to amputate Donna's leg. She was just that blunt. She said she wanted to wait a while because if they did it now, they would have to amputate above her knee. It was asked if they could just remove the foot, by this time it was black.

Someone mentioned to Donna's surgeon that her fingers were turning shades of blue. She bluntly said, "And then they would have to go the way of the leg." I remember thinking, "Oh heck no!"' From that point, I started massaging her fingers and hands. Everyone just sat there numb and quiet. Donna's surgeon just lets everyone soak in everything. She stated again that she hoped she only had to amputate below the knee.

Marcy: *the morning after Donna's transfer to the second hospital, we drove there. I remember arriving and hoping those who were already there had some news. There didn't seem to be anything that gave hope.*

The first morning in the step-down unit when her breakfast arrived, understand that Donna had had no solid foods for days, maybe even a week. I pulled the lid off, and it was a full breakfast, eggs, toast, bacon, juice. Of course, I was livid! She could hardly hold her head up — how was she going to eat real food? She couldn't hold a fork or a piece of toast. She could barely swallow. I talked to the nurse. It was crazy. Then the occupational therapist came in; he tried to get her to sit up, and swing her legs over the edge of the bed and stand up. Really! She couldn't do it, but knowing her determination, she certainly tried. He helped pull her to her feet, but it was obvious even to him she couldn't hold her position. Donna was too weak and mentally was foggy on his commands. She had been moved too soon. Critical care beds are few, and they try to free them up for more-critical patients, but Donna was not close to ready for this.

It had been a long morning, and I thought she could swallow something soft, so I asked if she wanted ice cream and Donna said yes. I ran downstairs, got soft serve, and began feeding it to her. It was a slow process, but she was getting something in her. She ate some but was done. After a bit, a nurse came in with medication in pill form. Again, I was shocked! I thought Donna isn't going to be able to swallow those. Well, the nurse saw that, so she said she'd put it in applesauce. So, I stepped out as she asked and she fed the applesauce, and Donna began to choke. It was crazy! Over the loudspeaker, they paged her room number and some code. It was insane! I stood outside her door looking in as they worked on her. A black middle-aged female custodian was cleaning the hallway. She slowed her work and hung back a little. She called me over to her. She said not to worry; Donna would be okay. She had seen it before when someone choked on food. She'd be praying for Donna. The problem was she didn't know how bad Donna had been and how bad she still was. They called to return her to ICU, where she should have been kept in the first place.

Somehow in the second ICU room, things seemed worse, bleaker. The urine bag stayed practically empty, and any urine in it was dark, very dark. Once again Donna's hand (or hands) began to turn purple. All I could think was, God, she can't lose her hand too!!!

From the last day at the first hospital through a few days before I left the second hospital, it was apparent that Donna would have to lose her foot, but the doctors weren't saying anything about it. I was concerned that the toes had turned black and that gangrene had set in, which would increase the risk of the infection traveling through Donna's bloodstream or system.

It was almost time for me to leave and I didn't want to. I had no one to keep the kids and had no choice, but

*I recalled not being sure if I'd ever see or hear or touch
Donna alive again. It was a gut-wrenching time.*

Having my family and support system there as things
started to spin out of control was vital. They were the
ones persistently pressing the doctors for information, my
Mom, Nettie, Alisha, Adrianna, Carolyn, Marc, Annie,
Cindy. When I was coherent enough each gently helped
me understanding all that went on.

5

PULSE CHECK

———◄◆●◆►———

*It doesn't matter what you've gone through in life, the
door on life did not close on you. You have the power to
rise above whatever you went through.*

— Donna Hopkins

very traumatic situation is tough on everyone. Sometimes what you go through isn't always for you, but
for those who are looking on. The only responsibility that is on your shoulders is how you go through and
come out on the other side.

It's hard for me to recall much of what transpired for
those three months starting in June of 2010. It's all a fog;
most of the time I was in a world of the unknown.

After taking some time to recover, both physically and
mentally, I decided to read over my medical records and get
together with my family and friends who were there with
me, to fill in the blanks. It was difficult reading my files.
It made me see for the first time just how close I came to

death and how terrible and scary things got. The real evidence was through pictures a friend had taken. I looked like I was hanging onto life by a thin thread or less. All those machines that I was hooked up to would have made anyone lose hope. Beyond the pictures, my family and friends gave me a distinct in-depth look into the darkest hours of my life.

Each of us was trying to make sense of what happened and how something that was supposed to have been simple went so wrong. In this chapter, my friends and family will tell you my story through their eyes. Cindy, Annie, Marcy, Nettie, Alisha, and many others will take you inside the walls of the hospitals, where we all awaited answers.

> Cindy: *It reads like it happened to someone else. What I learned broke my heart, but then I moved on to knowing that Donna was going to be okay and functioning maybe not exactly as before, but well. If this was emotional for all of us, I wonder how she felt when reading what happened.*
>
> *[While Donna was at the second hospital, the Los Angeles Lakers were in the finals of the NBA playoffs. The Lakers are Donna's favorite NBA team.]*
>
> *I cannot believe that Donna and I are having a conversation about them, being that she is delirious but lucid enough to know the Lakers were playing and she was watching them on television. I wondered if it was registering with Donna, because she had me by the arm and she was whispering, "Shhh, Cindy. Cindy listen, the Lakers have to win." I said 'Okay Jean," and Donna said, "No, no, listen, the Lakers have to win this game." Again, I say, "Okay, Jean!" Donna looked around the room—that's why I knew she wasn't all there because*

Donna was looking around the room like spies would jump out, and she said, "Shhh, the Lakers have to win!" I remembered thinking that I couldn't believe she was talking about a freaking basketball game! That's when I knew she was a real Lakers fan!

Marcy: *When her hands started turning purple at the second hospital, I told the medical staff the purple tinge and not having much feeling was how the foot began, and how ultimately, she was going to lose it. They examined the hands. I am not sure what they did—perhaps increase the blood thinner medication. I don't know.*

The most devastating moment was when I looked at Donna's eyes, which by now would barely stay open. I saw the whites were turning yellow, a dreaded sign of liver failure. If one foot had to go, at least there was the second foot. If one kidney went, she still had the second one. But I knew once the liver shut down, it was all over. And now the liver was shutting down. It was the most terrible feeling. It seemed everything was going wrong.

I remember everyone, even me, taking great pains to keep Donna's foot covered so that she didn't see it until she was strong enough. As her urine output continued to darken, I recalled a conversation with the medical staff as they considered putting her on dialysis. Because she was never stable enough to take on the stress of dialysis, they postponed it, and thank God; they never had to do it.

Some of the worst things I saw at both hospitals. I could say the worst thing I saw at the first hospital was the discoloration of Donna's toes, but it was the deterioration of her mental state and the rapid decline of her health. At the second hospital, I will never be able to erase from my memory the most shocking thing. Things got worse, but this was most shocking: I think they would only let us in Donna's room one at a time and when I went in, no one warned me, but she was so swollen, her body had retained so much fluid that even her eyeballs were swollen. They were swollen so much that when she closed her eyelids, it wouldn't cover them. I knew then we were in big trouble.

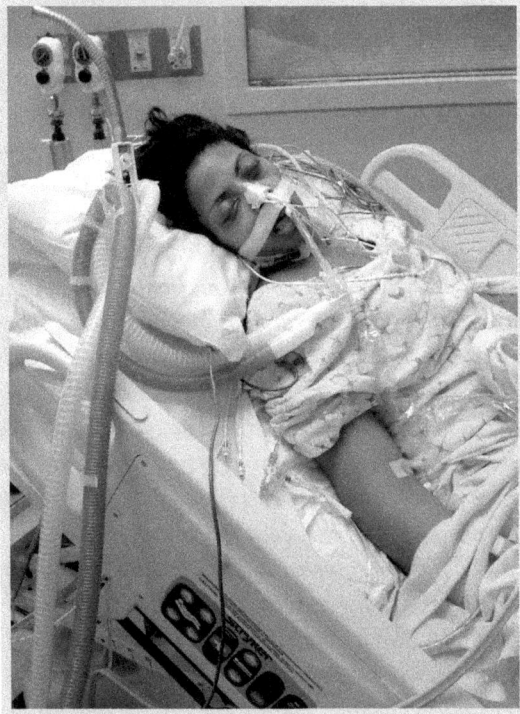

The other bad thing was the "elephant" in the room. We were all focused on saving Donna's life because she was so near death. We were so focused on saving her life; it was in God's hands all along. We watched the monitors, her oxygen levels, and the poor quality of her urine output, her blood pressure, her labored breathing and sometimes in-distress heartbeat. We all wanted more than

anything for her to live, but always in the back of our minds was the foot. It had now changed from purple to black. I knew it couldn't be saved, but we said nothing to her. I knew gangrene would or had set in and, in her teetering condition, continued to express concern about it getting into her bloodstream and taking her out.

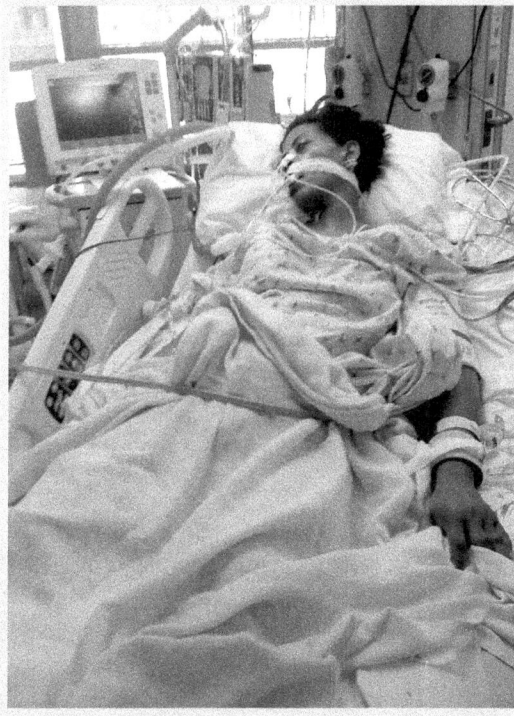

The other evidence we were in clear trouble was when Donna had water bubbles, like big blisters the size of quarters, full of water, popping up on the surface of her skin. I had never seen anything like that in various areas of her body. The doctor told us that her body was so swollen that when it couldn't hold anymore, it would

seep out just under the skin. Then there was the watching of the urine bag. To me, it was getting darker and darker with less and less volume. It was evident Donna's kidneys were failing, but the staff didn't seem to want to say that. The communication was so secretive, I think they knew what they were doing, but trying to keep her alive, or at least turning the boat in a better direction, was tough. And they didn't want to say.

After the water bubbles, they thought Donna was doing well enough to move her to a step-down unit, which provides an intermediate range of care for patients who are not sick enough for ICU but too sick for a standard private room. I didn't think that they should be moving her to the step-down unit, but they did. They said an occupational therapist would come in daily to help her sit up, stand up, etc. I for sure knew she wasn't ready to be standing up or much else, she was still too weak.

It was summer, and I came from California with no coat or jacket. I'd try to sleep when I returned to the waiting area, but it was freezing. All I could do was shiver. The next day I ran into a couple in the waiting area who said they saw me shivering. That's how cold it was. I remember them coming into the waiting area worried about their loved one. They later told me she had died — not what I needed to hear. It was evident we were in the worst-case ward.

In the ICU, rooms were going down one corridor with the nurses' station across to monitor. The room immediately to the left had a guard stationed outside, as did one more or so rooms down the hall to the right. I had never seen that before but found out that both were prisoners/convicts, and the one to the left had suffered a major heart attack requiring heart surgery. It felt like a little added security having a guard there considering the prisoner room was next to Donna's.

Then there was the flashing episode. I had come through the doors of the ICU. Once through the doors you still had sixty or so feet to go to get to Donna's room. As I came through the doors, I could see the prisoner's guard had angled his body toward Donna's doorway, looking in, he was trying not to be obvious to the staff, but it was so obvious. He didn't see me coming because he was looking so hard at Donna. When I got to her door, I knew what had captured his attention: her boob! The hospital gown had come untied at the neck and slid down Donna's front. I pulled it back up and told him he should have the decency not to look! After I had told the nurse on duty, they moved his chair to the other side.

Donna had started to become physically active, trying to get out of the bed, trying to take the tubes out. Cindy said the other night she was trying to take the hospital gown off because she was warm, and then she went for the central line in her neck. They wanted to restrain her, but Carolyn and I asked if one of us would stay with her the whole time, would they not tie Donna's hands with restraints. When one of us was with her, and a nurse came in to change her IV/monitor or change sheets or do something that would take a few minutes, we would take a quick bathroom break.

During one of my nights, a nurse came in. She and I chatted. She told me she was an ICU visiting nurse and that she and her husband drive across country in an RV. They plan their routes to stay in certain cities for a few weeks. She then can work at a local hospital. There was no reason to doubt her capabilities, so I went to the bathroom. When I returned, she was flustered.

She said she had laid a pair of scissors on Donna's tray and Donna had picked them up and cut one of her tubes. Sad to say, Donna's hands were put in restraints after that. The next morning, I asked to see the nurse in charge and told her about the nurse leaving scissors. Apparently, a dangerous weapon where Donna could have easy access was even more hazardous because Donna wasn't in her right mind. Donna was still defiant, physical, and a bit mean. I remember telling the nurses how nice she was. That was stupid!

Cindy: *Donna is in good spirits, suffering from "ICU psychosis," when a patient is sick of tubes, needles, and hospitals. Oh yeah, she's tired of it. She'll want us to do something, and if we don't, she'll roll her eyes and turn her head away from you. Marcy says she reminds her of a puppy's hurt feelings, and that's just what it's like. With the meds in her system and the sleepiness, Donna talks out of her head. It's funny sometimes, like her trying to get me to go behind the nurse's back to give her ice water when she couldn't have it. She wrote a note to me to go to the other nurse and get it. Then she wanted Marcy to take the bindings off her hands, and when Marcy told her she couldn't, she turned her head away a little peeved. We all tried not to laugh.*

Marcy: *Carolyn was also ever-present at the first hospital. I knew she had been staying over, so on my first night there, I convinced her to get some sleep, and I'd stay up all night. Not sure if she wanted to because she was very protective of Donna. By then Carolyn was so tired, her body accepted its offer, and she slept, she woke up when they checked Donna's vitals and went back to sleep.*

    I have vivid memories of Nettie at the second hospital sitting there very self-contained, arms folded. Nettie would tell me about her conversations with God that she didn't want Donna to hurt or suffer and although she wanted to be selfish and keep her around, if it were his will to take her, she would accept it. Again, another sign we were in trouble. She, Cindy and I would sit shoulder to shoulder or as tight as possible in space. We always had to be touching someone. It was a crazy time. So glad in the end she made it through this adversity.

6

LIGHT OVERPOWERS DARKNESS

————◄◆◆►————

Deep faith in God brings a steadiness in life's greatest crises to be an overcomer.

— UNKNOWN

Cindy, *June 24, 2010: Donna is back, lucid, and asking questions! She's been in the hospital now for 22 days and asked her Nettie if she had a disease. She had no clear idea of all that she has gone on. Nettie told her, "No, you didn't have a disease; you had a horrible reaction to a medication that was used." She later asked me what the medication was and I told her. I told her she has taken us on a ride; she just shook her head. I told her so many were praying for her and she smiled. She spent some of the evenings gently talking to us and checking email messages and had asked Nettie for her cell phone (uh-oh!), then she promptly went to sleep a little after midnight. Nettie and I tiptoed out of the room and went home.*

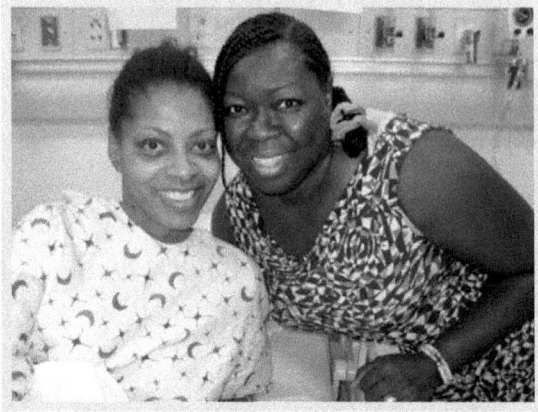

Cindy, *June 30, 2010: Can you believe that Donna was talking about the trip to Greece and she was saying she looked forward to it? Nettie said, " It's July 16," but she meant July 18. Donna said yes, and then I said, "You know July is two days away, " and then she understood. Tears welled up in her eyes, and she asked Nettie, "I won't be going to Greece, huh?" Nettie said "no".*

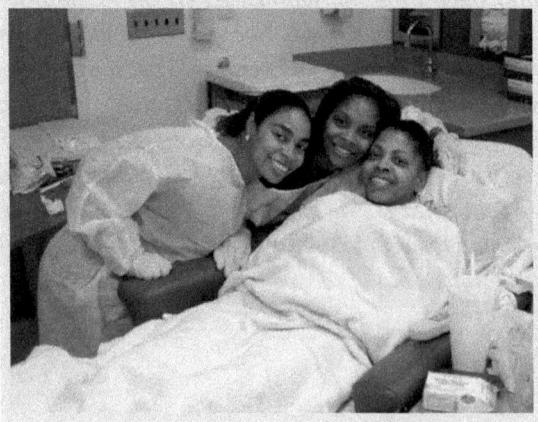

At this point, Donna has started speaking coherently; we were all glad. We could look into her eyes and see that she understood that something serious was going on, although she didn't entirely know what at that time.

Cindy, *to Donna: the surgeon had called in the family to stand with you while she spoke with you. The surgeon began telling you things that had happened when you arrived at the second hospital, the shock trauma hospital. The doctor said that you had to have your leg amputated. You understood what she was saying but you just looked at her, like something wasn't connecting with you, and then you looked at Nettie. You two just looked at each other and had this entire non-verbal conversation with each other. It came across to me like you were asking her if this was real and was it the only option for you being sick. You must have looked at each other about 30 or 40 seconds, and then you looked at the surgeon and nodded your head 'okay.' In those seconds of looking and searching, you understood that Nettie, that all of us, had done everything we could to try to save your leg, but this was the only answer to keep you alive and well. There was a collective sigh in the room.*

On Wednesday, July 7, 2010, the day before my amputation, I wasn't sure what I was feeling at this point; I think it still had not registered completely yet. I was still trying not to think about the amputation, and what all that would mean going forward.

The day of my surgery, July 8, most of my family was
there: Carolyn, Tonitta, Nettie, Adrianna, Annie, Lillian,
Cindy, Nettiel, Dru, Dewayne. My brother Roland had
come in from Detroit with my nephew Corey and niece
Sommer, and Sister Joe from the church was there. The
doctors were performing the amputation of my left leg
below the knee. That morning we started with a prayer, Lord
knows I needed everything to go right. Lillian, my sister,
led prayer and Annie gave me some blessed oil as I prepared
for surgery. Everyone went down with me for surgery; I had
my mini army, the front-line fighters. My doctors went over
everything with them and told them that surgery would take
about three hours. I kept my brainwaves free of any passing
thoughts concerning my surgery and what was about to take
place. I showed no emotions, one way or the other, to my family.
I was somewhat in a stage of being a vacant shell of avoidance,
trying to escape this unthinkable tragedy.

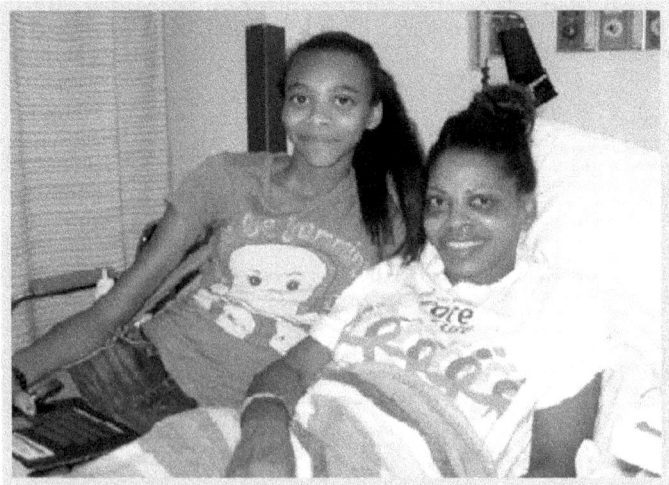

Cindy, *July 9, 2010: Donna is doing fine, after her sixth surgery yesterday morning, Day 35. She had the am-*

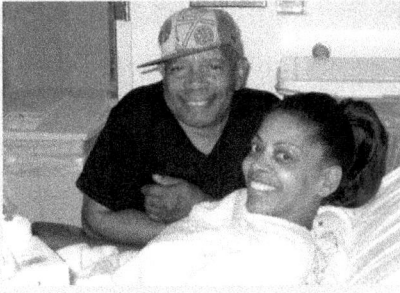

putation of her foot and partial leg about seven inches below the knee of her left leg. Many still do not know about this and Nettie, her family, and I are letting her tell it to others in her own time unless Donna asked us to relay it to someone. Donna left for surgery after prayer at about 8:30 a.m. and told us, " It's in God's hands, and I will be alright." Donna said she was ready to move ahead to the next stage. The surgery took about three hours, finished just before noon. Donna returned to recovery, and we could see her every two hours, two people at a time. She was in horrible pain at the beginning until they could manage it. She returned to her room just before ten that night, was wide awake, then just dozed off. The surgery team stopped in to check on her and woke her up, and the surgeon mentioned that all went well.

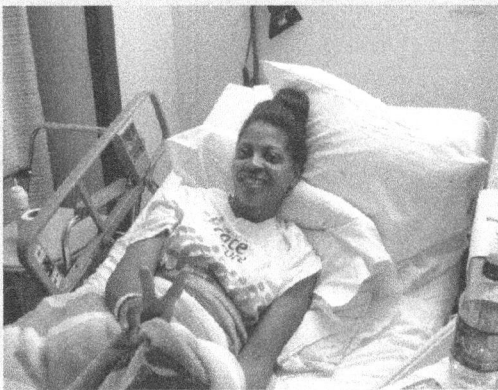

Now that death had finally taken its hands off me, I was on the upswing and soon would be released. Hallelujah! I could finally breathe life's fresh air again. I was still stuck in the hospital a little longer, however; my blood was being stubborn, and the levels would not cooperate with what the number was supposed to be.

Cindy, *July 12: To update you, C Ray, he is still to be glorified, even through all of this, her very life is a testimony to His goodness; she continues to say, "I am His!" She's touched many in her family. With the way Donna has handled this situation, she's touched my heart. The Lord continues to work things out for her, and that is encouraging, and she has her life.*

Cindy, *July 14, 2010, 2:05 p.m. (email to Marcy): I didn't want to upset Net, or you either, but I had to share this with someone. Life can change in a moment, I could cry, probably because I'm so tired. More likely, I'm in some weird melancholy-type mood. Her strength is coming back.*

Nettie, *July 14, at 2:41 p.m. (email to Cindy): Wow! It does not even seem real, and I know it is because I have seen it with my own eyes. Life!*

Cindy, *2:46 p.m. email: It makes me just say, "My God!" I wish I could go back to June 3, and kidnap her for the day; window-wishing again, I know. I guess at some therapeutic point; our minds will wrap around this for the long haul; because it's Donna and our lives now. Maybe it's the weather and fatigue that has me at this point, sorry to drag you guys along with me. No, I'm not; need you guys along with me.*

Nettie, *2:53 p.m., e-mail: All I can say is 'wow' with tears in my eyes.*

Cindy, *2:58 p.m, email: Me too, that's why I'm going to stop.*

It was July 15, and between the two hospital stays, I had been within hospital walls for 42 days. I was so ready to go home. My sister Carolyn was back with me as she had been, most of the time a welcome face when I woke up throughout the day. That morning, she started washing me off. I told her to go easy, that she was rubbing my skin too hard and that I could take over. I looked at myself, noticing how small I had gotten, and she confirmed that I was skin and bones. It was true; you could see my ribs. We both started laughing. The muscles that I had worked so hard to develop for years had evaporated.

As I turned my cell phone back on, all I could hear was the ding-ding of messages and calls being received. As I listened to and read them all, everyone was wondering where I was. There was an obvious concern in most voice messages since it was so unlike me not to return calls.

When I started calling some of my friends back, my nieces Nettiel and Dru laughed at me, saying I should have braced everyone before bursting into, "I went to the hospital for surgery for uterine fibroid tumors and ended up having to have part of my left leg amputated." I told them there was no flexible approach or easy way to let people know what happened.

Talking was challenging. My throat was hoarse, and my voice was a whisper, coming and going. The tubes down my throat had damaged my vocal cords. My friends were in disbelief as I described my story. I could almost hear their mouths drop on the other end of the phone, and I could only envision the look on their faces. Some of my friends were surprised at how I was handling the amputation of my foot and all that had happened. One told me they were talking to each other and crying but then thought to themselves, "Why are we crying? She's not."

Not knowing or understanding all that I had been through, I was just happy to be alive. Although I was out of the woods, my family was still protective of who could visit me, allowing just a few of my close friends. One of my good friends, Ellen and her son Justus came to see me. I thought it was great because, with everything that had happened, and him being young, he wasn't afraid, which made me feel good. He challenged my mind in games of checkers and tic-tac-toe. His competitive drive kicked in while mine was still in slow mode. My brain was still playing catch up.

Now that I was getting better, it was hard getting through the days in the hospital. Each day was the same: watching television, doing physical therapy, more TV and napping.

I still couldn't go outside, but on Sunday, July 18, they finally let my family take me out of my room for a while.

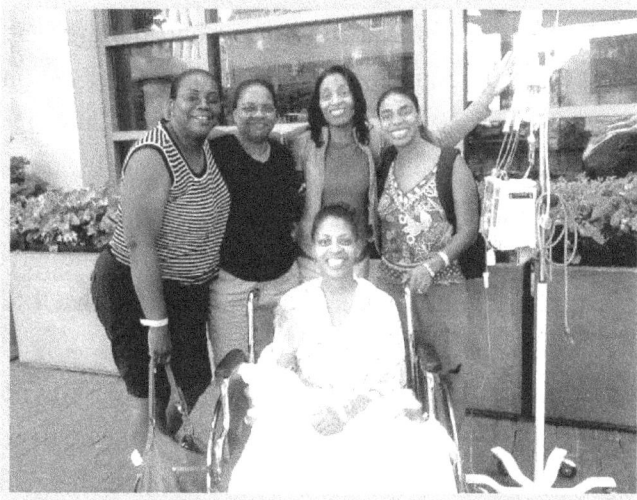

I was in this big oversized wheelchair, and my small-frame body looked like it was being swallowed up. There was room for two people to get in with me. As they wheeled me through the hospital, I was excited, combing my surroundings and taking it all in. For weeks, all I had seen was four walls and the same faces coming in and out of my room.

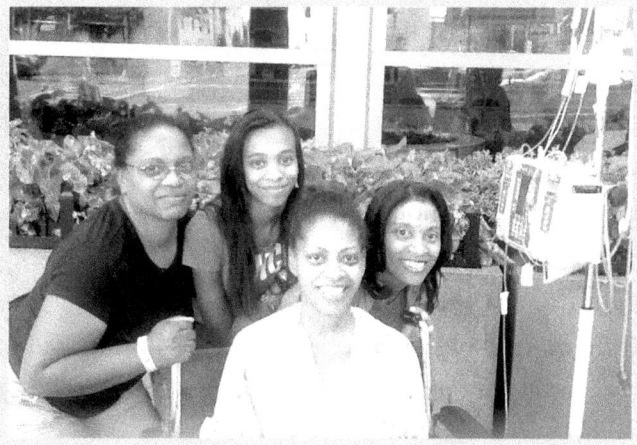

Although it was humid and boiling outside, they had a blanket over me because of my blood issues, and I was only outside for about 20 minutes. Nettie, Carolyn, Cindy, Dru, and Nicole were ecstatic, maybe more I was. Even with the heat, it was refreshing. It was good just to have the sun hitting my face. The summer was disappearing and, given my love of this time of year, I couldn't believe that I had missed most of it.

I had been in the hospital for a long time, and it was now time to get back to the stuff of daily life. None of us had thought about attending to any of those mundane things like bills. We had all been focused on me not dying. I guess the good part is I couldn't buy anything. I had missed out on all the summer sales, but on the other hand, I had also saved money. Nettie had forgotten to pick up my mail and so had missed the due date for my condo fee. That meant I had to pay a late fee. I should have written them a letter explaining things, but I went ahead and just paid it. Considering that I had been in the hospital so long, something was most likely going to fall through the cracks, but overall, we had been on top of the other bills. I'm glad that I wrote down my passwords and IDs to get into my accounts because at this point I could not remember anything, not even my home phone number.

On Thursday, July 22, the doctors told me that I was getting out the next day to go to the rehab hospital. My blood had finally reached the level they wanted, and these were sweet words to my ears. I had been in the hospital for 50 days.

On the 51st day, July 23, I thought that I was going to be released from the second hospital, only to find out later that I wasn't leaving. Thomas, my brother-in-law, was there with me. I get dressed around 2 p.m. after the caseworker told him and me that I would be released at 3 p.m. To my surprise, they came back in and said that, although the bed at the rehab hospital was ready for me, somehow the paperwork had not been completed.

I was dejected. I almost started crying. The caseworker left and went back to the rehab center. She called me later with more bad news: not only would I not be released, but now my release would be delayed until Monday. My face dropped. I pleaded with her to see if there was anything she could do. She called me back and said that I would be released on Saturday because they had worked something out. I was still a little distraught that I wasn't leaving that day.

Later that evening Nettie came up to visit, and we talked about prosthetics and life after losing my leg. She told me I was amazing and said, "I know you are a fighter and there are many things you are yet to do. Having a prosthetic will not slow you down. Once you get it and get adjusted to it, we won't be able to keep up with you. You were my inspiration before you lost your leg and even now without it, and I love you so much! My HERO!"

I began to cry because her words were better than any medicine for me at that stage, and she was speaking life into a catastrophic ordeal.

Saturday, July 24, 2010: Finally, I was leaving the second hospital, after 52 days. One of the nurses on the floor came and got me around 10:50 a.m., and it was so quick that my niece Alisha (who was with me) had to call Nettie to come pick her up. They loaded me on the bed and moved me out. I had a huge smile on my face and I couldn't believe that I was finally leaving.

I said goodbye to all the nurses who were there that had taken care of me and asked them to say goodbye to the others. Everyone had been great in caring for me.

So, we were off. I started texting and calling to let everyone know not to come up to the hospital. You would have thought that I was going home versus the rehab hospital.

Once I finished texting, I close my eyes. But it was refreshing to see everything on the ride down to D.C. and I wanted to see it. When we got to the rehab hospital, and they took me out of the ambulance, the worst heat hit me in the face. But I didn't care. I was one step from going home.

In talking to one of my doctors at the rehab hospital, I said that I almost died from heparin-induced thrombocytopenia (HIT). Nettie and Cindy told me about the blood clot that was in my left upper shoulder and was cleared up at the second hospital. They gave me some details of what had happened since my mind and memory were finally back to normal.

On Monday morning, they didn't waste any time getting me up for PT. They brought breakfast around 8 a.m., and I had to hurry through it since PT started at 8:26 a.m. Each PT session lasted half an hour. The first person had me remember a sentence and count from 20 backward. I thought, "It's not my memory that needs the PT."

On Tuesday, August 3, 2010 — 63 days after entering the first hospital — I finally went home! Sporting a thinner body than the one I came with. I walked on crutches down the hallway to my unit, with my sister Carolyn next to me.

We ran into some of my neighbors, and the look on their faces clearly showed their questions of, "What happened? We haven't seen you for a while." As I explained with the short version of my disappearing act, I told them it was the result of a medical disaster; they were speechless and stunned. I was still mystified at all that had happened, too.

As I walked through the doorway, I looked around, just happy to be home. I breathed in and out, grateful for each breath as I stood there for a moment, taking it all in. I took my time, so my thoughts could process the emotions that I was feeling to be home and, more importantly, alive.

I realized that I had just come through an incredible, horrendous life-changing experience, where the brakes had been put on my life for what seemed like forever. At this moment, I had to allow myself time to slowly take off the emergency brake so that I could exhale and move forward with the other part of my healing.

What did it all mean? I wasn't sure, but finding out had to be a minute-by-minute, hour- by-hour, and day-by-day process. I knew that I had to take my time to go through whatever process I needed to go through to deal with everything.

For me, it was about endurance, resilience, and fortitude, not a sprint race. This was a marathon during which I had to take my time, take in all my surroundings and figure out how to move forward in every aspect of my life.

My first step was not to look ahead because I didn't want my brain to be on overload trying to process too much or get frustrated thinking about what was ahead. So, for now, I just needed to ease back into being home.

My clothes were falling off me, nothing fit. My butt was reduced to a little bump and the muscles that sculpted my arms and legs were now just skin and bone. Carolyn had stayed behind with me since I couldn't travel yet while the others went home to West Virginia for the family reunion, something I had planned on attending before everything happened.

As I sat down on my couch, it was a welcome reunion of a different kind, just as it was while sleeping in my bed later that night. I felt a little lost, like a stranger in my own home. As I looked around, it was like I was seeing things for the first time, while also glad to see them again. Everything in my vision was refreshing and uplifting. I sat there as my eyes searched the room, gazing at each picture on the walls and all the things that were in the adjacent rooms.

Carolyn and I watched a little TV until I got tired and finally retired to bed.

In days to come, as I begin to live in my home again, I wanted to try and do some things on my own. Although I was still in the early stages of my recovery, I wanted to learn how to carry food or drink from the kitchen to other rooms while on crutches. Carolyn wasn't going to be with me for much longer, so this was necessary. I got some plastic grocery bags and containers with lids and carried my food and utensils that way. Most of the time I tried to get everything I needed because I didn't want to get back up. Trying to figure it all out was a little overwhelming at times, like getting in the tub, getting out, but the most challenging part was having to think about each time I got out of bed and had to put my foot down, or I got up from sitting in the chair. I couldn't just jump up and go that was disturbing and testing. I didn't like that feeling; it was something that I had to learn how to handle.

What helped me keep a positive perspective on what I had been through was jumping back into the things I enjoyed, as well as was my attitude about life.I didn't sit around crying but was spending more time with my family and friends, who help me stay upbeat and moving forward. One day when I was sitting around, I thought about some of the dark moments. At one point when I was in the second hospital, I felt like I had died. I could hear people talking like I was going to be missed. I heard my family, and it seemed like they were making plans as if my life was over. It was like I was looking down at them while they talked.

You must love family and friends and understand and excuse their heightened emotions, especially when something so inconceivable happens and death is so close. Everyone is afraid! I realized that my family and friends had gone through something too, even if they weren't the one lying in the hospitals fighting to survive life's darkest hit. They had their own struggles to overcome. They saw everything in full force and the impact it had on everyone throughout the long ordeal.

We all needed time to grieve; we needed time to slip away in meditation to quiet our aching hearts and souls. We needed time to flush our minds of an unwanted experience for which none of us signed up. We needed a renewing time, a quiet time to reflect and to sift through the memories and come to grips with what had happened to me. All of us needed the time to just cry for ourselves, because the devastation we all felt affected each one of us in so many ways. Our emotions had been at an all-time high, our strength had been shaken to the foundation, and at times our faith had been put in a furnace where the heat was intensified.

As we all escaped to our solitude, we had to find ways to pull ourselves through this difficulty. It became a time just to be who we needed to be when we each could open up ourselves to God and let the reassurance of His everlasting love start to heal our brokenness and bring a long-awaited peace to our souls. As I look back and recall the actions of my family, friends and myself, none of us allowed our spirits to be broken, although at times I'm sure there were cracks in our armor. For me, as I was in my world, too sick to realize all that was going on, God's ear was never too far to hear my inner cry for help. In the darkest hours, God's heart and mine became one as His heartbeat took over for mine to pump life back into a broken body.

7
THE PROCESS

————◄ ♦ ● ♦ ►————

*The making of each one of us happens in the process of
going through. A new level of who we are happens in
the process, healing comes in the process, all to help us
to move forward to victory.*

— Donna Hopkins

t is common for anyone to experience extreme emotional reactions when going through something devastating and shattering. To get to the other side of victory,
I had to go through the process, allowing myself the time
to mourn the losses I had experienced, recognizing this was
a challenging time, a day-by-day process.

At the end of August in 2010, I had my post-op appointment with the doctor that removed the fibroid tumors and
did the hysterectomy. Nettie and Alisha went with me; they
ended up asking most of the questions because I didn't know
much of what happened, other than what they had told me.
I sat there listening, trying to process all the information of

what was said. I think I was somewhat in a haze like they were all speaking a foreign language about someone else.

The more the doctor went over things, the more I started second-guessing my decision. Maybe I should have had the hysterectomy from the outset, but he said the same thing might have still happened. I sat there thinking to myself "I guess we will never know." I asked a few questions, but I was perplexed and therefore, didn't leave feeling good about all that I had heard. It made me question my decision, even more, considering the results. I smiled on the outside, but I cried within. I wished that I could have rewound the clock.

I knew that this doctor had a good heart and was saddened about what happened. He was still flabbergasted by all that occurred, and so were we.

To get out of the house, my sister decided to take me to the mall. I went to a couple of stores, but ended up parking my wheelchair in one section of the mall. I didn't feel like moving around in the wheelchair, so until my family returned, I watched people walk around freely, thinking, "That used to be me." It made me want to leave. I didn't let on to my family when they returned, because it was just something that I needed to work out within myself, and I didn't want to be more frustrated talking about it or start crying.

Carolyn and I then went to a movie. Since I was in a wheelchair, I had to sit up front, and I felt like the screen was hugging me in the face. By the time I left the movie, I had to do neck calisthenics to get the crick out of it.

In the process of moving forward, the gym has always been the medicine for my healing. Carolyn took me there. I wanted to get back to some sense of normalcy. When we got to the gym, I told her that instead of using the wheelchair, I wanted to use my crutches to walk in. Friends at the gym were happy to see me, and others who didn't know what happened were stunned. They said it was just like me to want to come to the gym and they conveyed that they would be there to assist in helping me get back on my feet. I told them I would hold them to it.

In weeks and months to come, I relied on some of their expertise to work on strengthening and improving my body's walking gait. I also shared what they had me doing in PT so that I could double my daily workouts. I was doing everything I could to get stronger and build my body back up so that I could quickly get back on my feet to walk again once I got the prosthetic.

Annie was thinking ahead for me; she had already arranged with the department of motor vehicles for me to get a handicap placard parking permit. I had no patience or tolerance for sitting around. I was eager to get moving again. I started driving about a week after getting out of the rehab hospital, whether I was supposed to or not.

Before I left the second hospital, my family and I had started looking at prosthetic companies. Once I got to the rehab hospital, one of the doctors who came to visit me was an amputee, and she told me about a few companies. She selected one from Florida. There was no way I could consider a Florida company with the financial burden of my medical bills and how often I would have to travel to Florida (for measuring and fittings) if I chose them.

I wanted to deal with a company that serviced the military and wounded warriors, and there were so many military bases in the Washington, D.C., metropolitan area. I knew this type of company would have more experience getting people back up on their feet, particularly since members of the military had seen so many war-related amputations in recent years.

I was doing some work at the Bethesda Naval Medical Center in the Morale, Welfare, and Recreation (MWR) sports department, and someone told me about one of the prosthetics companies at Walter Reed Army Medical Center. I went to meet with a representative to gather some information, and, in fact, he had his own company, Medical Center Orthotics and Prosthetics in Silver Spring, Maryland. That would be convenient for me since their office was about five minutes from my home. I made appointments with two companies. Although I had not visited MCOP's office, I had talked to Mike Corcoran, one of the owners.

I thought that I was just going for a consultation with Mike, but he started measuring and casting me for my first prosthetic. When I left, I thought, "What just happened? It was only supposed to be a meeting." I told myself this must be the sign to go with this company. I was surprised how fast things were moving. I got out of the hospital in August, and it was just September, and I was already getting fitted. I thought that it would at least be three months or more before I was ready for my new wheel. I guess my leg was healing enough to move forward.

For the past 20 years or so, I had covered the Washington Redskins for various outlets, currently "Tony McGee's Pro Football Plus" TV show. This NFL season wasn't going to start off exactly as I hoped. In fact, it would be entirely different and challenging, both physically and emotionally. Although many of my NFL official friends and some others had already spoken or seen me, I knew that many others in the media would be shocked and have many questions.

Training camp had already started at Redskins Park, and I wanted to go. I was still in a wheelchair. A lot of people would probably have closed themselves off from the world for a while if they had been in my situation, but I wanted to do things that I enjoyed, and it was also a form of healing for me. Going to camp would be a big step for me, facing everyone for the first time, them seeing me in a wheelchair, with part of my leg gone. I didn't want my face to give away that I was feeling emotional. I was a little shaky with them seeing me this way, and it made me somewhat uncomfortable.

When Carolyn and I first arrived at Redskins Park, coming into the building, I met a friendly face: one of my friends who is an NFL official was working at camp that day. I think what made me nervous was that I didn't know how everyone would take seeing me this way and how they would feel. It was hard for me to see myself this way.

After practice, I talked to Chris Samuels, a friend who played tackle on the offensive line for the Redskins. As we were talking, Gary Clark came up from the field. Gary and I have been friends since he played for the Washington Redskins in the 1990s, and we were currently working on "Tony McGee's Pro Football Plus" TV show. We always joked around with each other.

Chris was sitting in front of me, which hid my left leg. Gary saw me and was getting ready to rag me about being in the wheelchair until he walked around and saw my leg. That's the first time I saw the cat have his tongue. He was stunned after I told him what happened, he said had it happened to him he wouldn't be able to handle it, and he would be so mad. Funny, a lot of my friends said the same thing and stated that they would still have had the covers over their heads. My thinking was that I had already survived death, and it would have been a tragedy to die emotionally and physically after what happened.

Once the pre-season and regular season started, Carolyn, Nettie, and Alisha accompanied me to games to help me get in and out of my truck with the wheelchair.

When I went back to work in August, many people dropped by my cube to say hello or talk, but a friend, "City" Michele Fisher, made herself my office police. She kept people away or ran them away because she didn't want people overwhelming me in my first few days back.

After being in the office for a few weeks, my division had a luncheon for me so that everyone could welcome me back. My niece Alisha was close beside me as the other office police.

Although I appreciated the outpouring of warmth and kindness from everyone, one thing that stood out for me at the luncheon was a poem that one of my co-workers and friends Sherri Cook wrote:

SHE GETS IT

Donna is truly a survivor – SHE GOT IT.

This life deals us a hand we cannot trade back with the dealer; you see the winners in life learn to focus on just achieving.

Conquering those trying times in life is a skill.

Donna has a spirit that displays sheer determination and faith.

Many of us have seen struggles; many of us have had to climb mountains, so you understand when I say Press On. Donna has proven to us and will continue to show us just what it means to Press On and not give up on that hand dealt.

Emotionally, spiritually, & physically she gives it her all 100% with a real commitment. This luncheon is also for all of you and me.

As individuals, co-workers, mothers and fathers, daughters and sons, aunts and uncles, we can learn a great life lesson in dealing with that hand dealt. Recognize what you have to figure out, which way you want to go, set a game plan, and head in the right direction.

There may be players (roadblocks) that come across your table, but that's okay. It happened to help you rethink your game plan, your strategy, but never changing the goal to win, achieve, succeed.

DONNA GOT IT…WE ALL NEED TO…………
GET IT

Sherri Cook
08/2010

CELEBRATE LIFE!!!

Sherri went on to say, "It will take some time to transform ourselves from a loss to living victoriously, no matter what has happened to us. Given the right inspiration and passion, like her, we all will get there." I tried to fight back the tears, but those words filled my heart with joy, and at that moment it made me realize the almost-death experience I went through wasn't for nothing. I got it. It spoke to my life survivorship over the years; it made me appreciate and understand it myself. You never know who is watching and what your life speaks to others. My niece comforted me as I wiped away tears, fighting to control them.

In early September, I was at work sitting in my truck at lunch, and I was watching people pass my truck. I found myself watching people walk a lot more, looking at their legs. I thought to myself: we take things for granted like walking, running, and our eyesight. We never believe that anything will happen to us, and when it does, we appreciate the time when things were different.

Later that day, when riding home, I was so uncomfortable. Sitting for extended periods of time with my leg hanging was uncomfortable because I hadn't gotten my prosthetics yet. My emotions were all over the place because my hair was coming out by the handful due to all the medications that I had been taking for the past few months. I was coughing all the time, and my voice was hoarse most of the time. So, as I drove home, I wanted to burst into tears. I think it was just one of those days when everything just hit me.

On September 6, I went home to West Virginia to visit and check on my mom, and I don't think I moved off the couch much. They brought my food to me. My niece Alisha told me, "You are not helpless." I told her I was somewhat limited for now.

Ever since I got out of the hospital, it was hard for me to stand to wash my hair, so while in West Virginia one of my sisters decided to help me. What a disaster. As Lillian washed my hair, I was thinking, "what kind of washing is she doing?" She was splashing water in my eyes. I felt like a child again when my mom washed it.

My hair was so tangled; I had to take over. I got under the dryer to condition it — another mistake. It was like a ball of confusion on my head. It knotted up even more. It was like a yarn ball, and as I tried to get some of the tangles out, it was a lost cause. It was a mess at this stage. It had locked up on one side. I looked like I had a unicorn horn on my head.

We went to Walmart to see if we could get hair products to get the tangles out, but we had no luck. I immediately called my hairdresser back in Maryland to set up an appointment and explain what happened. He said I could see him right away when I got back. I was shaking my head in disbelief; I was in dismay thinking, "now this?"

My sister Lillian was saying she was sorry, but I just shook my head at her. I knew this wasn't her fault; it was a result of all that I had been through that had weakened my hair. My family tried to make me feel better, saying it will grow back. At that point, I wasn't feeling what they were saying; I just saw my unicorn head.

When I got to my hairdresser, he tried to work out the tangles but to no avail. He stated that he had no choice but to cut my hair. I looked at him as if my eyes were saying, "tell me anything but that." As he started to cut away, he tried his best not to cut much off, but my hair was in bad shape, falling out and tangled. I never had short hair before. As he started to cut it, I watched each piece fall to the floor, wanting to pick it back up to salvage each strand. I didn't say anything, but my heart was feeling it, like being hit with a blow each time a strand fell to the floor. It probably really wasn't about the hair, which had to be cut off, but more to do with everything else at this point.

At this juncture, I surely didn't need anything more to happen. I wanted to cry, but I told myself, considering what you just came through, this was minor. In the days and weeks to come, my hair started falling out more, I looked in the mirror and could see bald spots. My hair was so thin you could see right through it; the bald spots were visible throughout my entire head, my once-long hair that had draped down my back was barely a frame that shaped my head. I decided I would get a wig because I wasn't comfortable with my hair being almost gone, and for many reasons it made me feel better.

Early on, you could see God's hand in the restoration and therapy process. He always has a ram in the bush as our lookout. For each person who will ever have to go through anything traumatic, God knows what we need to get us to the other side of victory. Alisha had been in an Under Armour store and when in the checkout line, she was drawn to a card and picked it up. Little did she know how this would be an aid and inspiration in my healing overall. Under Armour was gearing up for its 2011 "Power in Pink: She's a Fighter" campaign to celebrate women's' courageous fight against breast cancer. They were looking for three breast cancer survivors to celebrate the many women who use fitness and exercise to stay healthy and serve as a platform to help raise awareness about breast health.

The campaign was Under Armour's fifth annual survivor search in the United States to help raise awareness of the importance of leading a physically active life in the fight against breast cancer. So, to honor, inspire, and support women who were fighting breast cancer, Under Armour was encouraging survivors and women currently living with breast cancer to share their stories of strength and survival on their website. They were going to select three stories of courage and hope from women who would become the new faces of the "Power in Pink" brand campaign, and continue to empower and raise awareness of the vital link between physical activity and recovery from breast cancer.

As a part of its national campaign, the selected winners would receive an all-expenses-paid trip to Under Armour headquarters in Baltimore, where they would be part of a photo shoot and awarded $5,000 for their charity of choice. My niece thought this would be worthwhile and valuable for me in my recovery, and right up my alley to tell my story about how sports and fitness had been the medicine I have used to get me through every suffering or difficulty.

I only had a day or so to write my story and get it posted on the Under Armour website for approval. Also, for the first time since the initial launch of the campaign, consumers were going to play a part in the selection of the three survivors in a "fan favorite" section to be voted on by site visitors. On September 13, 2011, Under Armour announced that I, along with Erin Stone and Erin Taylor, was selected in its fifth annual "Power in Pink: She's a Fighter" search. We would share our stories of inspiration on a national scale as the faces of Under Armour's "Power in Pink" brand campaign.

As I wrote in chapter one, it is amazing how things can hit you in life that you never expected would come your way, and how these things will change you and your life forever. In my Under Armour essay, I said that I was a sports lover and had used sports as my escape as I went through treatment and recovery.

I knew that my attitude and positive outlook on life had a lot to do with me surviving. What got me through cancer twice was my unrelenting faith and my love for life. I always say, "What doesn't kill you makes you stronger." Had I not gotten breast cancer, I would never have started a foundation in 2000 that helps breast cancer survivors.

I told Under Armour that I was indeed the winner in everything that I've gone through, and I stand with the gold medal of life. Being selected by Under Armour as one of the faces in their 2011 "Power in Pink" campaign was truly the remedy that I needed at that moment. It helped me in the process of getting me through the amputation and its aftermath. It was like God had dropped a gem of happiness and joy out of the sky into my lap.

A friend emailed me after hearing about my association with Under Armour. She wrote, "I just had the chance to read your story and watch your UA video. I think I had told you before, back in the day when we worked together at the blues, I believe that you are one of, if not the most beautiful person inside and out that I have ever met. It still holds true today. After all, you have been through, nothing ever broke your spirit or your faith, and after watching your video, you inspire me even more. You are one awesome woman, and I am thankful that I have the privilege of knowing you and calling you my friend. You go, girl!!!"

I think that, behind whatever you must go through in the process of living life, you are the one that controls the way others will remember you, by the way, you lived. And it is God's light that can shine through any darkness (John 1:5).

Thursday, December 13: I started my quest to make the Paralympic team in wheelchair basketball. I was training with the men's team, who were soldiers at the Walter Reed National Military Medical Center. I met the coach and informed him of my plans to try to make the Paralympics. He stated that he would put me on the men's team to get me ready. He noted that it would be hard going against the men, but it would get me ready when I played the women. I told him I had played with male players before this all happened. I played mostly with men in pickup basketball, and I had played college basketball. Wheelchair basketball is a whole different challenge, but I told him I was up for it. I was in the gym every day working to strengthen my upper body, because being in a wheelchair and shooting foul shots, I couldn't even get the ball to the rim. Can you say, "air ball?"

It was a little frustrating not being able to do some of the drills. It was harder than I thought, trying to operate and control the chair, dribble, and shoot, among other things. I wanted to be able to play like I did when I played upright. I had to tell myself this was just my first day, but my competitive nature kept kicking in.

They said that on Wednesday, December 19, the men's basketball team from George Mason University would be coming to play us. It was exciting "playing" against George Mason University's team. They were in for an eye-opening experience. Their basketball talent and skillfulness were about to be put on center stage. They quickly realized that playing upright was much different than controlling and playing in a wheelchair. In the wheelchair, you are only allowed one push, and then you have to dribble the ball.

As we zipped past them, we looked like we were the Harlem Globetrotters with all the tricks that made their heads spin. After getting on the court in wheelchairs, they had a greater understanding and appreciation for just what it took to play in a wheelchair. They appreciated what we had overcome.

We then played in a tournament at Fort Belvoir, with both amputees and soldiers from the base making up the team. It was an experience playing against other teams that had played for years, but we held our own.

I also ended up playing and practicing with a wheelchair basketball team out of Washington, D.C., under Coach Bill Green's leadership. Although I never traveled with them in tournaments, I enjoyed practicing with the team on weekdays and Saturday mornings.

In December, I headed home to West Virginia by train because the weather was bad. I went home to spend Christmas with my mom. She had been through a tough time, in and out of the hospital, and now she could not walk and needed someone with her at all times. I was still on crutches because I had just gotten my prosthetic leg a few months back. My sister Adrianna picked me up at the train station. The weather was bad as we drove up the mountain.

Once I got to the house, I didn't move out of my dad's big blue chair the whole time I was there. That night,

Christmas Eve, I was in the big oversized chair, and my mom was on the couch. We watched my sister Adrianna, and her daughter Alisha put up the Christmas tree. All of us ended up sleeping in the living room that night watching the Hallmark channel's Christmas movies — Alisha on the love seat, Adrianna on the floor next to our mom, me on the reclining chair, and my mom on the couch. I was only there for a day and a half, but I was glad that I could go home. I never watched so many Christmas movies in my entire life, but just being able to be there was such a good thing. In fact, it ended up being my mom's last Christmas, so I was happy that I could spend it with her.

In January 2011, we had an ice storm. I never liked the cold or that time of year as an adult, and even more so once I was an amputee. I was heading out to work after a two-hour delay. I could not imagine going out in the dark to face that ice; it was bad enough in the light. As I looked outside, I could see that my housing development hadn't yet cleared any ice.

However, Annie had stopped on her way to work and removed the ice from the front and back windows of my truck. I should have stayed home; it would have been the logical thing to do. As I headed out on the slippery surface, I called it my unwise journey to the treacherous pursuit of something that wasn't going to end with me upright.

As I walked out of the front door of my building, I was looking at the ice on the ground. For about three minutes I wondered how I was going to get across the ice to my truck. I stood there waiting for someone to come out, but when they did, I just let them go right by me. I used my crutches to get started, digging them down into the ice. I was already at a disadvantage and to top it off; I had on sneakers. I was asking to fall. I got to the middle of the roadway between the building and my truck and got stuck.

I looked around hoping that someone else would come out. I dug the crutch down into the ice more, and my right leg slid. I was thinking, if I go down, I'm never going to be able to get back up. So, I stood there, rethinking my decision, but at this point, it was too late. A guy finally came out; I thought about asking him if I could hold onto his arm to get to my truck, but my mouth stayed closed. I don't know if it was because my brain had stopped working, or my independence had made me stupid.

I was back on my own, so I used my crutches almost like ski poles to dig harder into the ice. Finally, I made it. I needed to shovel the area between my truck and the car next to me to get out. I started to go back in, but that meant tackling the ice again to get back to the building. Next time, lesson learned: stay home. I ended up just getting in the truck and driving to work.

As I struggled to find my new identity and confidence and comfort with myself, I was learning how to accept who I was. In the process of moving through the amputation, some people saw a form of healing and opportunity for me that I didn't see for myself at the time. What is vital is finding out what keeps you moving forward. Sports and competition have always been medicine for my soul. I was doing physical therapy with someone that a friend had recommended, outside of my regular physical therapy at NRH. This person worked in the amputee clinic at Walter Reed with soldiers who had lost limbs. Adele was like the hidden light, shining my way, directing me on this new path.

I started working with her at Walter Reed. I found out that she also lived close to me, so I reached out to her, and she said she would help me with my PT. Even though I was going to PT at NRH, she added a different component. Adele would draw on paper the exercises we did so that I could do them at home on my own. Each time I came back, she challenged me in new ways.

Not too long after working with Adele, she suggested I get into rowing. She said I could compete to go to the Paralympics in Rio in 2016. I told her I couldn't swim; she told me she would teach me to swim or I could wear a life jacket. I told her I would think about it, but even if I was not sure about it, I couldn't pass up a good challenge when it came to sports. She told me when the rowing coach would be back at Walter Reed. I eventually went to meet the coach, who was recruiting soldiers who had lost limbs at Walter Reed.

Lucky for me, because visiting that day was a member of the 2012 U.S. women's Olympic gold medal eight-person rowing team who competed in London. I thought that I was just going to talk to the coach and was not dressed to row, but he put me on one of the rowing machines and took me through a few drills.

The Olympian had her gold medal. Many wanted to take pictures with her holding it, but I asked if I could put the gold medal around my neck so that I could feel what it would be like when I got my own. We then took a picture together.

The coach informed me about the program and invited me to practice with others who were involved in the rowing program in the spring at the local boathouse. Adele was more excited than I was at that moment. Her will was going to get me to Rio. She also told me that summer was coming soon, and I would be able to show off my leg, but I thought to myself, no, not ready yet. I was comfortable in my long pants covering up my leg.

On Sunday, March 13, I got a call from one of my sisters that we needed to get home right away because my mom was sick and in the hospital and they weren't expecting her to live. I called my other sisters and nieces in the area and told them that I was getting ready to pack up my stuff and get on the road to go home. When I got to the hospital and walked into her room, I saw all the monitors. She was hooked up to a ventilator and in distress.

I wanted to burst into tears, but I fought them back, trying to stay under control. I bent over and started talking and praying for my mom. I told her we were going to be all right, and then God dropped a song in my spirit to sing to her that seemed to calm her down. I knew it was the end. She had been suffering for so long with one illness after another, and at this stage, she couldn't walk or take care of herself, and she didn't like that. Adrianna, Alisha, and I stayed the night while the others went to our mom's house.

Early in the morning, a nurse came into the waiting room, woke us up, and told us that we needed to call the others because there was nothing else they could do for our mom. My sister Adrianna called and told everyone to get there. Walking into that room, I could see on her face that she was in such distress. I believe she was holding on, struggling to make sure we were going to be okay. I told her that we got this for her now and that all of us were going to be alright. If her assignment was over on this earth, it was okay for her to depart.

My niece was overwhelmed, rightly so, and I told her she needed to tell her grandmother that she was going to be okay. So, she did, crying. Adrianna was standing with tears coming down her face. I fought back the tears. I told myself I needed to stay under control, and I knew if one tear came down my face, the gates would open.

I was sitting holding my mom's hand; they put her back on the ventilator to calm her breathing because she was struggling so hard to breathe. I was holding her hand and looking at the heart monitor as her heart rate was going down. I cannot get the picture out of my head as I watched the monitor flat line. I thought it was a movie I had watched, but now it was a reality for all of us; it was a throb and sting. My heart was evaporating with pain from watching her in her last moments before death. As everyone else got there and entered the room, I left and went back to the waiting room. As I walked out of that room, I wanted to run to a place of escape, but also knew that strength must kick in not just for me, but for everyone else, since they were falling apart.

I had just watched my mom pass away. It was the hardest thing to see. After the nurses cleaned her up, they asked if I wanted to go back in. I said no, I didn't want to see her that way. They told me she just looked like she was peacefully sleeping. Still, I didn't go back in; I was still trying to get the image out of my head, of seeing her struggling to breathe and then die. It was painful, gut-wrenching. I went into my private bomb shelter to protect myself from the emotional fallout surrounding me. Once everyone got back to the waiting room, I started planning her funeral. I was numb. I couldn't cry, although I wanted to. There wasn't any time because everyone else was filling the river of sorrow with their tears, and that was okay. I couldn't because I promised my mom that we had this, so I moved into action.

I stood up for the family at her funeral by writing a tribute to her. One of my sisters said I wouldn't be able to do it without breaking down. I knew it was going to be hard, but I went into my secret place of strength and pulled off the shelf what I needed to sustain myself. I told my sister I had to; I wanted to make sure that our mom's life's work was rightly reflected. To us, she was a beautiful mother, grandmother, aunt; a mother to many, the anchor, the glue that held not only our family together but those of her siblings, being that she had been the last one still living out of 19. I told myself I had to stay strong, it was vital. Her life spoke so much to so many down through the years.

I never had the time to escape into my solitude, to mourn my loss some months before. I had to conceal my pain to face another type of pain. After burying my mom, my heart ached.

Outwardly I had to be strong, a strong face that I had to wear most of my life. I had to hold back the tears I wanted to release while I allowed others to express their pain about our mom's death.

There came a time when I wanted to cry and couldn't. There was no water coming down the river; it was a drought of emptiness and disconnection. If you cannot release your pain, "a desert will form, and the rain of liberation — the rain that brings comfort and restores life—will seep through the cracks." You cannot be a force of strength for everyone else and not have the water flowing back to you; otherwise, it will cause you to die.

8

TAKE THE MASK OFF

◄ ◆ ● ◆ ►

*I learned that courage was not the absence of fear, but
the triumph over it. The brave man is not he who does
not feel afraid, but he who conquers that fear.*
— Nelson Mandela

A t times, the emotional side of everything that had
happened would resurface, and questions came
flooding in. I asked God what this was all about.
Was there a reason or purpose my leg was amputated? Is
there something I'm supposed to learn from this?

What happened to me in 2010 was so overwhelming in
so many ways. I had to ask myself, did I pray before I went
into surgery? Did I ask God to watch over me and cover
me and to make sure that nothing went wrong? Considering what took place, I thought I must not have. Nettie told
me not to question or wrestle with my decision because I
made the best decision with the information I had. I knew
she was right; I had to let it go.

I had spent so much time adjusting to walking again, getting back to competing in sports, and being busy doing other things that I hadn't dealt with the other side of the amputation: the emotional and psychological adjustments. You tell yourself that you are good, or that you will be alright, but inside there is a clash between your emotions and the physical side of things.

Each time I passed by a mirror, I didn't want to look at myself. I would quickly look away. I tried not to be mad, but it was a reminder of the 2010 impairment. There were times I looked at my life and thought: Will anyone want me now that I am an amputee? People are so quick to look at the surface. I knew what was imperative was learning how to love myself again. I was so worried about how others would see me and treat me after the amputation. I realized that this was more about how I saw myself.

It's surprising how we assume that the physical is more detrimental than the emotional. Don't get me wrong, having my leg gone was injurious, but it is the emotional side of things that is like a massive, unrelenting weight.

After the amputation, I didn't want to spend a lot of time being upset or in a dark place about what had happened to me; it was vital for me to get back to living. What should have been equally critical was slowing down and confronting and dealing inwardly with what had happened.

I finally took the time to search my feelings. The storms of turmoil had reached a point as David describes in Psalms. I cried out to God, how long will you wait until you come to my rescue? Where are you? Are you ever going to change my situation? Clouded by all that had happened, God was there; I just needed to pay attention and not look for signs in the traditional way. God was there working behind the scenes. He was the master carpenter, carving and making and putting the broken pieces of my life back together again.

The first step was to stop replaying in my head the footage of what had occurred in the hospital. Even though I had come through breast cancer twice, along with hyperthyroidism, this was different. The challenge was different, and the emotions were, too.

After being out of the hospital for some time, my focus was getting out of the wheelchair and being able to walk again. The rest of 2010 was spent getting my strength back, getting fitted for prosthetics, and learning how to get around physically with my new outfitted device.

In the beginning, it was challenging, as my mind and body were in dispute with each other.

Getting used to the prosthetic was awkward and weird. Early on, the pressure was intense because my leg was still healing. It was uncomfortable; it felt like I was dragging along an extra load. I felt like my body was cut in half, one side normal while the other side always felt off balance and somewhat disconnected. I had this whipping foot motion when walking because my quads and glutes weren't strong enough at first. At times, I was frustrated, and it was a struggle. However, over time as I got stronger, physically and mentally, it got better, it just became part of me, but still, never like having my real leg and foot.

2011 was more about just recovering: doing physical therapy, learning to walk, getting my new leg, and dealing with the death of my mother. I jumped right back into everything — gym, work, covering the Redskins, foundation, church, you name it. These things helped with my healing, to some degree. I still hadn't taken off the mask.

I believe there is a process that we all must go through if there is going to be complete healing, restoration, and renewal from the brokenness to repair our mind, spirit, and body. I realized that more and more.

I remember a message that Sister Leslie Bishop Joe had spoken at a women's retreat I had attended: God will meet you right where you are. I needed God to meet me where I was at this point in my inward struggle.

I believe that, no matter what happens to you, you can find something that inspires you to keep going. I got involved in rowing in 2013 with Coach Patrick of MedStar National Rehabilitation Hospital's rowing program. Adele, my physical therapist at Walter Reed, had suggested it to me. The first thing I told her was that I couldn't swim, but she said she could teach me. I agreed, but when I thought more about it, I thought I must be crazy even to consider it. At the time, I was considering what sport I wanted to train for in my quest to make the Paralympics in 2016. Adele thought that rowing might be it.

Before the outdoor season started, I met up with the rowing coach at Walter Reed and informed him I would give it a shot. The first time outdoors on the Anacostia River, not being able to swim was on my mind, but the coach was yelling so much I didn't even have a chance to think about it. I thought I must be back in college with my basketball coach. I was thinking, "Gee, this is my first time on the water, and he is yelling like that." All I wanted was for him to go work with the other individuals in another boat.

That day, after being on the water, I wanted to run for the hills. I thought rowing was not for me. However, I went to the gym the next day to try applying some of the things I learned at practice on the rowing machine. Although it was not the same as being on the water, I could still work on some of the technical skills the coach had pointed out.

My second time out, I was surprised when the coach informed me that I was going to be in a doubles boat race the next day. I was thinking he had to be kidding; I needed to be a little more comfortable. I was so nervous the day of the race, but I had a great teammate who told me that, even though he had two more races after ours, he was going to put everything into our race because we were going to win. It was a little windy that day, which made the water a little choppy and rough and made me nervous.

I decided not to wear a life jacket. Later, Cindy fussed at me after she found out I didn't wear one. My teammate Wesley told me as we got in line for boat number 4 to do what we did in practice the day before. I was in the front of the boat; Wesley was the lead in the second seat. He said we needed to get off to a good start to get ahead and stay there. We began with a "power 10," power strokes so that we could make a move at the start and get out in front. I slid off the seat and had to readjust. It was a 1,000-meter race. We had a good start. There were four boats in the race. We were neck-and-neck with one of the other teams' boats, but we pulled ahead.

Sometimes I lost my form but got it back. Ahead of the other rowing boats, Wesley was in my ear the entire race, pushing me, because at one point I was so tired. But he yelled out, "You are not tired." Yes, I was! He told me boat three was getting tired. After we had gone under a bridge, he wanted us to push the last 50 meters. I had to dig deep because at that point my heart was beating outside my chest and my legs were fatigued and stinging. I dug in, along with him yelling out directions for another power 10, still telling me I wasn't tired.

When we went across that finish line, I had nothing left, nothing. It was Wesley's coaching that got me through; he was great. Unbelievably, we got first place. It was such a good feeling. Coach texted me later and said he was impressed that I came away with the gold medal on my first time out. I thought maybe that was a good sign. My teammate Wesley was a high school junior.

At the race, some other people were talking to me about wheelchair basketball and tennis, but the rowing coach told them to stop trying to take his recruits. That was race No. 1 of working toward the Paralympics. Rowing was good because I didn't have anything to measure it by, it became a source of therapy, treatment, and renewal to rebuilding. It took me to a place of victory in some areas that I needed.

When I told my family and friends about my quest to make the Paralympics, they were excited and thrilled for me; all of them said they were booking their ticket to Rio de Janeiro, Brazil. I think they were just as excited about the thought of me trying to go as I was, but most of all, they were just happy for me. I loved the fact that some of my friends and family came out to watch me row, they took pictures and cheered me on, which meant a lot to me. I wanted them to experience this with me. I could hear them yelling, "go, Donna, go." Those who couldn't come to watch me compete would always call or email me wanting the results, and when they heard them, they left the most encouraging messages. One friend even helped me when I decided that I was going to try to make it in track, he had run himself in high school and college. He worked out with me, giving me feedback on my running techniques, among other things that were helpful.

It took about a year, but in 2013 I started to settle back into my routine. For my family and friends, they were there if I needed them, but they allowed me the space to go through the process in my way and in my own time. I realized the physical part of me had gotten back on track, but when I re-examined my inner self, I discovered some unresolved feelings that I had buried. As much as I love God, I realized that part of me was upset with him for not stepping in and preventing all of this from happening. Why at this stage of my life? Why at all? I'm an athlete at heart, an energetic person full of life. He knew me better than anyone. Wasn't it enough that I already had two bouts of breast cancer and thyroid disease? Was I to be a living Job? I was thinking; I already took my hits for the kingdom. Down through the years, all I had heard was, "God wants the best for you." Well, this surely couldn't be the best.

I thought back to that Bible verse where it says that God would not put more on you than you can handle, but always makes a way of escape so that you can bear it. Then I heard some of my friends say, "God knew that you could take it; otherwise he wouldn't have allowed it." I was thinking "I'm not trying to hear that." All I knew was part of my leg was missing, and that life was going to change totally. Some of my friends said that they would be angry for life. I was distraught, troubled, in a state of disbelief. I knew that I had to become bare before God, and strip off the layers; otherwise, I was going to be trapped.

I started thinking more about church and life and my relationship with God, and I saw it so differently since the amputation. For some time, even before my amputation, I had felt a disconnection spiritually. Some of it was on me, and some were with my unhappiness with "the church" and religion in general. Before I knew it, part of me had died spiritually, and the cry within me was seeking and yearning to relink with God and reset. But how? With all that I knew about God, I was in an empty place, where I couldn't pray or read the Bible to reawaken the fire. I knew that God was holding me in his secret place, and at this critical time, I was withdrawing my bottled-up pleas for help.

I was at a turning point in my life. I wasn't going to allow people to put me in a box anymore and make me think or act like they thought I should after coming through 2010. It was about God and me. The only opinion that mattered at this point was God's.

What I learned in the process of recovering is that sometimes our churches and people think that, if you didn't die after what you went through, you should be intact and ready to jump right back into things and move on. I heard a sermon where the preacher said, "It is one thing for God to deliver you out of that tragedy you went through, but what is going to propel you forward is for him to sustain you. When God sustains you, he strengthens and supports you physically and mentally so you can get past the devastation."

When I thought about my situation and how unexpectedly it all came about, I thought about a storm and how it comes and moves on quickly, leaving behind its destruction. The aftermath of the storm leaves you with the cleanup of trying to piece your life back together. The cleanup can be harder than the storm itself. When looking at life's storms, life's disappointments, life's frustrations, heartaches, tragedies, catastrophes, and misfortunes, they all cost us something, but it is up to us to determine if we want to recover or not.

After coming through a place of devastation and emotional anguish, I faced the underlying wounds confronting me. I wasn't sure of all that I was feeling; it was a lot to tackle, looking toward the future with the changes in my life. When taking off my clothing, I saw all my life's battle scars, but the most revealing was the internal scars that weren't showing on the surface.

The first step was learning to love me all over again and accepting that person. I didn't want other people treating me any differently, or looking at me any differently, yet I was doing just that. Despite what I looked like, I had to remember that I was still the same person, and a friend reminded me of it. He said that he wasn't going to treat me any differently despite my amputation because I hadn't changed behind all that had happened. Little did he know how much those words made me feel good; they did more than any natural medicine could do. It was healing to my spirit and soul.

A great comfort for me throughout my ordeal was that — even though my mom was sick herself and fighting to live — before her death, she was still there for me; a mother's love that was invoking life back into her daughter's body. I wanted for her what she desired for me: to live.

When I was in the hospital, I was already setting a goal on how to get back up on my feet and move forward. Slowly and steadily, sustained by my faith and support from family and friends, I took off the mask and reconstructed my life.

9

RESETTING

---◄ ◆ ● ◆ ►---

We can reset our lives as many times as we need to. As we each travel on our life's journeys, there is still a rainbow that shines a light to help us travel on the roads to wherever we set the navigation to. It is in reaching the end that we learn a little more about what makes us who we are and what helps us to move forward.

— Donna Hopkins

once heard the soul is our living presence. It is the one thing that cannot be altered. It lives despite how our body lets us down. Our body will let us down, but it's up to us not to let ourselves down.

One day in the early stages of my amputation, I was sitting in my truck watching people walk by, and thought, "That used to be me, just simply walking, nothing hard about it, no thought or effort to it, just putting one foot forward after the other." Now, walking is like continually fine-tuning an instrument. Once you figure out the right tone, it becomes a beautiful sound.

Susan Taylor, editor-in-chief of *Essence* Magazine, wrote something in one of her articles that resonated with me: "Whether a change delights us or makes us struggle, it always ushers in a new beginning. It forces us to be engaged in life, to focus, to give birth to new ways of being and to continue to open up our eyes to see, so that we may fulfill our purpose."

In June 2017, I had one track meet to qualify for the Paralympics trials in Atlanta, which would take place in early July. It was also the last track meet where I could get my Paralympics track and field classification, which I had to have to run in the trials. I had one shot!

With only four months to train, I had my work cut out for me. I had to shift gears from rowing to track. I thought that rowing would be my ticket to the games, but despite winning most of my races, getting selected for the team was difficult.

In 2016, someone had seen me run at a running clinic in Washington, D.C., and thought that I should consider trying out for the Paralympics track team. Since it was a sport that I had done before, I figured maybe they were right, so why not?

I started out working with a former high school coach who had coached my niece but ended up with a coach who had experience working with amputees since he was one himself. After my first workout, I questioned why I was taking my body through this brutality.

Every Saturday morning, I was at the high school track, pushing my body to exhaustion. I couldn't even let up, because my coach, who had his stopwatch, was yelling as I came around the track, "Keep going, push harder, get your knees up, drive!" Before I could catch my breath from finishing 130 meters, he was saying, "Let's go again." Running the 130 meters was done to strengthen me for the 100 so that I had power at the end to finish strong. The day's practice was eight 100-meter races, finishing with three 200s.

My body and mind were in a fight with each other, one telling me to stop, the other telling me to keep pushing, sometimes both wanting to walk away. My races were the 100 and 200, but Coach and I had decided that since we had a short window to get my body back into track shape, we would mainly focus on the 100 meters.

My warm-ups were just as grueling as the actual running. My coach would pull out all these gadgets to work on my footwork, race starts and getting my knees up for powering down the track.

This particular day we were working on exploding around the curves and picking up my knees going down the straightaway. My right leg with the running spikes dug into the track as I came around the curve. My coach called out, "Lean more into the turn." As I came to the straightaway, he told me to pump my arms more, and pick up my knees and drive. Sometimes my prosthetic side would hydroplane with the increase of speed, and I would stumble, almost falling. I needed to pick up my prosthetic leg more. By the time, I finished running those eight 100s and one of the 200s, I looked at the coach to say, "I have nothing left."

Before heading off to Chicago for the qualifying meet, at my final practice, my coach said we had done everything we could to prepare me for this moment. He told me to run and not think about anything else. I was a little nervous because he couldn't go with me.

My results: 0.33 seconds. That is how close I came to making it to the 2017 Paralympics trials in Atlanta. The competitor in me was disappointed and sad that I missed out, but in the same breath, proud of what I had accomplished in such a short timeframe.

I wish that I could draw the perfect picture for each journey in my life. Sometimes what goes into the drawing and the final version are not what we may have sought after or envisioned, but the finished picture can still be one of beauty.

In the wake of my misfortune, considering what I had gone through, I concluded that sometimes God uses the things that should have destroyed you to develop you.

Romans 8:28 reads, "We know that all things work together for good to them that love God, to them who are called per his purpose." Psalms 46:1-4 says, "God is my refuge and strength an everlasting help in times of trouble. We shall not fear though the earth gives way and the mountains fall into the heart of the sea. Though its waters roar and foam and the mountains quake with their surging and even if everything is collapsing around you and the unknown is no longer there we should have no fear because God is our refuge and strength. The more troubled the waters, the more God will be present."

Whether the Lord sends a trial or permits one to occur, he said he would use it as part of his plan for our good. Looking at the situation with our own eyes, it won't look too good, but the promises of God allow us to see it through his eyes and how he sees it. How do we get through (Psalms 103:19)? We must know that there's nothing that is outside of His control.

When difficulties come in our life, they can make us feel off course and unsure of our direction. When death hovered over me in 2010 and threatened to take me out, it was God's loving arms that pulled me through to the other side of victory. His hand was the light that shined through my darkness. I believe that, through it all, God was placing in me a testimony for all to see. I remember reading that if we trusted God's sovereignty that cares for us in life's storms, he would use us to bear witness to others.

When things are out of control, and at the most heightened time, God's hand reaches in to perform the cleanup from what we have gone through, to renew and rebuild. We only must go through the process that leads to the promise.

A friend shared with me a story about his neighbor. He said, "I was just thinking about you, and how it's never been easy for you and your health. It made me think about what a friend's son said during his father's funeral. His father was disabled for as long as I knew him. He started out with a cane, and then progressed to a wheelchair, funny that I used 'progressed' when referring to his disability. For as long as I knew him, he never complained about his situation. That was the theme presented at his celebration, and that made me think of you."

I thought about what he said in this email. The man could have protested his condition — he had every right — but he chose not to see himself as hindered or cast down despite his circumstance. That recalled a quote by Abraham Lincoln: "In the end, it's not the years in your life that count, it is the life in your years."

Some years after my amputation, I was at an event at the Kennedy Center. A soldier whom I had met at the gym at the Walter Reed National Military Medical Center had lost both of his legs in the Iraq war. He was receiving an award. In his acceptance of the award, he stated that an essential part of who he is was not the person you were looking at from the outside, but who he was inside. That resonated in my spirit because my heart made the connection to what he said to be true in my own life.

How did I plow through the darkest time in my life to find my light again? As I hit the reset button, I did my self-examination; I searched out what was broken in me so that I could take it to God. I realized it was through every tear I cried that healing came forward. Healing also came when I could completely open my heart to God, that he could come in and perform the emergency surgery that was needed to breathe new life back into every broken area of my life, physically, emotionally, and mentally. In God's great understanding of me, he knew what I needed so that healing could come forward.

I thought about getting older with the amputation and concern arose, but through it all, even if I didn't see the rainbow in my life as I looked to the future, God saw it for me.

I honestly believe that, while it might not be crystal clear why difficulties happen, they still have a reason that can work for our good if we let them. I was visiting a church one Sunday when something the pastor said caught my attention. He stated that sometimes you have no control over the storm; sometimes storms are essential and needed. We need to stop asking why, but rather look at how we respond during our adversities. He then stated, "We are not called to trust the results we want, but to trust God and his plan for us."

Ask yourself, what is the thing that lies at the bottom of your heart that beats life into you again? Find it! Transform yourself after something happens, and realize that happiness is not in someone else's pocket. You have the key — pull it out and open the door to your new beginning. Know that you are stronger than any pain that you must go through; you must tap into that hidden strength.

In my retooling of myself, I came out with a newfound outlook on life in moving forward. It is about taking life by the hand and running with it to wherever it will take me, and letting my hair blow in the wind as I move through each journey and undertaking. It is about making the most out of every day. I made up my mind not to be around joy zappers — people who cry all the time or complain about everything.

Laughter is such strong medicine that its effect reaches beyond any pill. It brings healing to the soul in ways that nothing else can. Learn how to surround yourself with good people who can make you laugh and will add joy and peace to your life.

Even when life slams you to the ground without any warning, know that in everything we go through, there are triumphs and victories. Sometimes God allows things to happen knowing that he can entrust us to carry out his assignment, not only for our life but in helping others in theirs.

There will be great losses in our lives, and many people will try to rush you through the process of moving forward, but take the time to mourn whatever the loss is and then move forward. Our time here is limited, so there's no time to waste by staying locked into the world of what happened. Don't allow what happened to you to rob you of your tomorrow.

The driving force in keeping me going was God and his purpose for my life. One thing I have learned is to live life to the fullest because one thing is for sure: everyone is going to die, but few will truly live. Live life to the fullest! You must decide what that means for you.

Despite what I went through, life is still great, and my new beginning will be substantially fulfilled, always with a joy for life. Many prayers went up for me, and I believe that it was those prayers that bent the ear of God to say, "Donna's assignment is not over yet." As each of us moves forward, God will calm everything until we can stand up on our own again, where we can face what we'll go through. As Isaiah 40:29-31 says, "He gives power to the weak, and to those who have no might He increases strength."

How do you find your way again? Take one breath at a time and allow yourself to breathe again. The heartbeat of who you are will be found in what you go through and how you come through it. It is OK to cry about your circumstances, the devastation, destruction, and adversity, but don't drown in your tears. Don't allow them to be the anchor that keeps you from coming up again.

I fought back with everything I had. Each of us must know that there is light at the end of darkness if you keep pushing through to see it. We all have the answer inside as to what it will take to carry us over to the other side of victory, but it is up to each of us to keep digging until the answer is clear.

Looking back through the lens of what I came through, I'm moving through what inspires me to push forward to live. The key to unlocking the door of what I went through was finding what inspired me to get through my pain, to cross over to the other side of victory.

There is no timetable for when you should be healed. It's a process, and everyone's process is different. The way I got to the other side of victory is not how you might get there. The key is to get there.

ABOUT THE AUTHOR

West Virginia native, Donna Hopkins is the 8th of 10 children born to the late Irving and Nazimova Hopkins. She is a graduate of Fairmont State University, where she earned degrees in Radio & Television Communication and Regents of Arts. An athlete at heart, she earned scholarships in both basketball and track. After college, she moved to the Washington, D.C., metropolitan area where she currently resides. Donna is a sports television personality, currently a co-host and reporter for Tony McGee Pro Football Plus on Mid Atlantic Sports Net (MASN), the author of *Getting to the other side of Victory*, Founder/CEO of the non-profit Hopkins Breast Cancer Inc., a public speaker for breast cancer awareness programs, an inspirational and motivational speaker, a two-time breast cancer survivor and an amputee. She is on a mission to share her triumphant journey and to teach individuals how to reset and tap into the hidden strength we all have, the passions and the purposes that drive us to not only win for ourselves but for others.

————◂◆●◆▸————

The making of each one of us happens in the process of going through, a new level of who we are happens in the process, healing comes in the process, all to help us to move forward to victory.
— *Donna Hopkins*

BLOG:
Inspire me today, your inspirational kick with Donna
DONNAJHOPKINS.COM/2017/05/25/FIRST-BLOG-POST/

DONNA'S WEBSITE:
WWW.DONNAJHOPKINS.COM

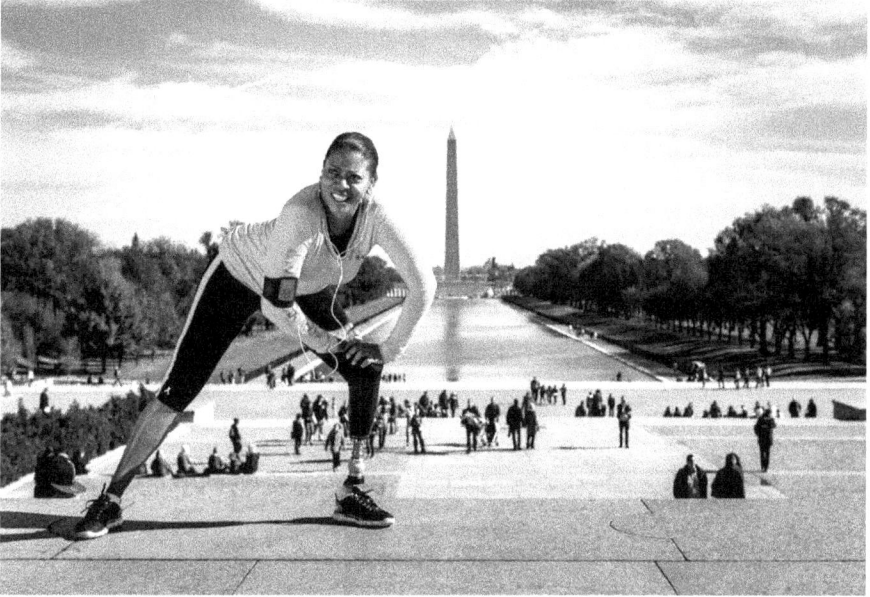

ÖSSUR®

*Helping people live a life
without limitations*

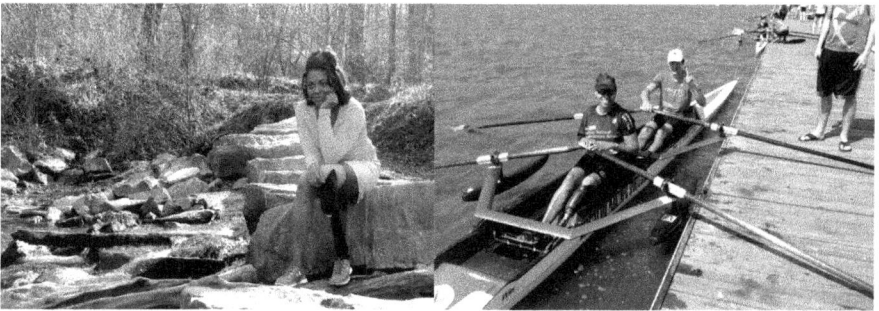

www.ingramcontent.com/pod-product-compliance
Lightning Source LLC
Chambersburg PA
CBHW060337030426
42336CB00011B/1378